P9-CMC-983

FROM HERE TO LONGEVITY

Your Complete Guide for a
Long and Healthy Life

Mitra Ray, Ph.D.

with
Patricia Cannon Childs

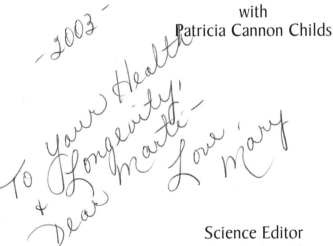

- 2003 -

To Your Health
& Longevity!
Dear Marti -
Love, Mary

Science Editor
Cynthia Sholes, Ph.D.

SHINING STAR PUBLISHING
Seattle, Washington

Copyright ©2002 by Mitra Ray, Ph.D.

All rights reserved. No part of this book may be reproduced in any form or by any electronic or mechanical means, including information storage and retrieval systems, without permission in writing from the publisher, except by a reviewer, who may quote brief passages in a review.

Printed in the United States of America.

LIMITED FIRST EDITION

Library of Congress Cataloging-in-Publication Data
Ray, Mitra.
    From here to longevity : your complete guide for a
    long and healthy life / Mitra Ray with Patricia Cannon
    Childs. -- 1st ed.
      p. cm.
      Includes bibliographical references and index.
      ISBN 0-9714842-0-4

      1. Longevity. 2. Health.   I. Childs, Patricia
    Cannon. II. Title.

    RA776.75.R39 2002   613
                                QBI02-200161

DESIGN BY JILL BYRD WILLIAMS

Shining Star Publishing
P.O. Box 85821
Seattle, Washington 98145-0821
www.fromheretolongevity.com

—for my mother and in loving memory of my father

Table of Contents

List of Figures

† Denotes figures that are enhanced in *Figure Reproductions* towards
the back of this book

To My Readers

One of the main objectives of this book is to redirect the dollars that you spend on your health. We all spend a great deal of money on items that impact our health, whether it be on junk food, pharmaceuticals and emergency care, or on organic groceries, free-range meats, food supplements and yoga classes. Here are two key points that every consumer should know:

1. Phillip Morris Companies, Inc. is now the second largest food company in the world. That means that you are buying much of the food you eat from a tobacco company.[1]

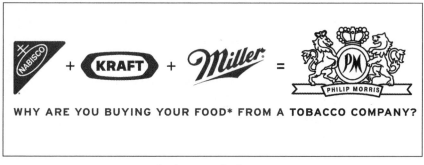

Courtesy www.adbusters.org.

---

[1] "FTC Approves Nabisco-Phillip Morris Deal," New York Times, December 7, 2000.

2. The laws of economics govern pharmaceutical companies. This means that it's more profitable for them to spend research and development dollars on maintenance products that treat the symptoms, and that people will use for the rest of their lives, than it is for them to develop products that treat the actual causes of disease. That's because the latter approach represents a one-time expenditure on the consumer end, which is not very good for business.

Since you're going to spend money on your health no matter what, the real question is whether you want to spend it on sick care or healthcare. I want to encourage you to redirect some of that spending—away from treating symptoms and toward the possibility of prevention.

I believe that it's time for us all to take more personal initiative and responsibility for the quality of our lives. I am also convinced that in the long run, when it comes to healthcare, this redirected spending will be more economical, both for us as individuals and for our society as a whole.

If I could financially profit from every dollar you spent on prevention, then I would be proud to earn that money. But it would be neither prudent nor possible for me to spread myself so thin as to represent every great thing out there that has the potential to help us lead healthier lives. Since this book is full of suggestions for books, products and services, I feel it is important that I tell you about any financial benefits that I might receive if you choose to follow any of my recommendations.

My husband and I have an independent distributorship with NSA, Inc., the marketers of Juice Plus+®. If you were to choose to buy Juice Plus+® from our distributorship, then we would make a small profit from that purchase. If you were to buy the product from another distributorship, independent of ours, then we would not make any profit. Our distributorship represents a small fraction of total NSA, Inc. sales. I have no financial ties to any other books, products or services that I mention in these pages.

In the course of this book, I'll mention some of the most important things that I've personally run across and use in my own life that I feel benefit my family and me. Moreover, the book should provide you with enough knowledge that, should you run into some other product or service that sounds good to you, you'll be in a better position to make an informed decision for yourself.

Happy reading,

Mitra Ray

Acknowledgements

How does someone take on the writing of a book? Only with the loving support and encouragement of her family, friends and associates.

I am grateful to all of the people in my life who have supported me in the creation of this book. I especially thank my husband for giving up sunny days of paragliding, sailing and skiing in order to be here for me. I also acknowledge my children, Leela and Nira, for being such wonderful inspiration and for reminding me of the world we are building for them. I thank my brother, Dipankar Ray, for a lifetime of insightful conversations and for the love and support he has always given me. I thank my nanny, Valeda King, for taking such good care of my children. I would like to thank Dr. Cindy Sholes and William Kennamore for their initial enthusiasm that kindled my imagination, and thank you Cindy for also being my Science Editor. Critical to the book's coming to fruition was Patricia Childs. Her integrity and commitment allowed me to remain inspired throughout the project. Thank you Jill Williams for your imaginative artwork and layout. When I had the nerve to ask my sister-in-law/English teacher Kelly Koffman to critique my book, her loving dedication to detail really brought this project together for me. And, Gillian

Riley, far away in England, giving up her valuable time to read and comment on each chapter as it was being completed, added an international flavor to the common issues we all share.

I wish to thank Ki McGraw, Bob Smith and all of the instructors at the Hatha Yoga Center of Seattle for their instruction and encouragement. My mind, my soul and my back thank you for the tranquil strength you've given to me.

I also wish to thank Landmark Education for opening me to a new way of being. Without the "Conversation for Possibility" I might never have seen myself as an author. Over the years, the courses offered at Landmark Education have continued to expand my sense of what is possible for human beings and for the future of our planet.

I want to acknowledge Dr. Richard DuBois, Dr. Barbara Fischer, Professor Robert Sapolsky and Leslie Montag for all of their support. And although there isn't room to mention you by name, I want to thank all of you who have invested in this project with your energy, your time, your encouragement and your love.

Helpful Resources

At the end of the book, *Suggested Reading* includes brief descriptions or reviews by Dr. Ray of books that might reinforce or supplement the ideas presented here. The section that follows is *Figure Reproductions*, which contains selected figures from the text that are re-presented here for further clarity. Finally, the *Selected Bibliography* contains the references cited in the text and it is organized by chapter.

Publisher's Note:

The information provided in this book is intended to help readers play a more active role in their own healthcare. It is not intended in any way to replace the services and expertise of trained health professionals, particularly with regard to symptoms that may require diagnosis and/or immediate attention.

lon · gev · i · ty

(lon · jev′ i · tē, lôn-) *noun*
1. Long, vital life. **2.** Great duration of life.
[Synonyms: health, ripe old age.]

1

So Many Questions

So, you want to become healthy. You get inspired and go to the health food store. When you get there, for all the money in the world, you can't figure out which supplements you should buy. What are the differences among them? Why was it that you thought you needed them? You have some vague notion that you need to take supplements because of an article you read in a magazine; but what about the rest of your grocery list? Should you buy non-fat milk or reduced-fat milk or whole milk—or, perhaps, soy milk or rice milk? Should you cut all the carbohydrates out of your diet as you read in that book last month, or should you eat according to your blood type as suggested in another book your friend recommended this month? Is there a quick, convenient bar that you can snack on this afternoon that is healthy, or is this the day you should start eating collard greens and kale? Is soy bad or good? Do you need hormone replacement therapy? Should you see a chiropractor? What the heck is homeopathic medicine anyway? And why in the world do people rave about acupuncture; how can it be fun to be poked with needles? Since you seem to be losing your memory lately, are you bound to get Alzheimer's disease? Or will cancer get you first? Should you take up walking or jogging or weight lifting? Maybe yoga and meditation are the way to go. How many minutes do you have to work out and for how many days to see some results? Should you fork out the bucks and join that gym; or are you finally going to watch those workout videos at home? Why is it all so complicated?

These are only a few of the questions that plague the minds of those of us who have finally realized that we are not invincible after all, and that we need to do something about our health. Then there are those people in crisis, who are faced with decisions about chemotherapy or radiation or surgery or holistic treatments. Others are trying to become pregnant or they are new parents, and they are struggling with balancing their lives, or wondering whether they should immunize their children. It's been said, "We are drowning in a sea of information, seeking knowledge."

In some ways we've made tremendous progress in understanding how the body works and in creating new biotechnology. Just think, we now have artificial pumps that help a failing heart to circulate blood through the body. Still, there are vast differences of opinion about what should be done to alleviate and prevent disease. Until recently, prevention was not even a major focus for the medical establishment; yet the combination of alarming statistics for degenerative diseases and rocketing costs for healthcare has forced mainstream medicine finally to shift its focus.

I love life. I want to live forever; but given that I can't

do that, I still want to live a productive, healthy and happy life for as long as I can. That's why I have such an interest in the topic of health. Even with my training, as a Ph.D. in Cell Biology from Stanford Medical School, I had difficulty making sense of all the choices I described earlier. When I was at Stanford, my thesis advisor was Dr. Lubert Stryer. He has written one of the most recognized books in the field of biochemistry; one which is used in medical schools all over the world. As a student of biochemistry, I gained much insight from this book. However, as a person who wanted to live a long and healthy life, I found a huge gap between the known biochemistry and its application. Why wasn't all of this knowledge being taught to everyone in a way that would promote health and longevity? I've also read many other books on physiology, molecular biology, cell biology and chemistry in a disappointing search for that connection. The book that I'm writing here is my attempt to bridge that gap—for me and for you my valued readers. This is not to say that there are no good books on health out there. In fact, there are some excellent books that I'll cite and recommend here for further reading. But the intention of this book is to bring together what I've found to be the most beneficial and practical information from my on-going research, and to focus attention on the current philosophy of healthcare. As we progress, I'll also offer viable alternatives to our current approach to health, both for individuals and for our healthcare system. The changes I propose are designed to promote a long and healthy life for as many people as possible, in a healthcare environment that actively supports that goal on a day-to-day basis.

How, you might ask, did I come by such a heady objective? Well, it occurred to me that every day there are more and more people who decide to travel the road to longevity. These people soon find themselves adrift in that "sea of information" I mentioned earlier. With a bookstore in every shopping mall and advances in communication technologies, we have almost immediate access to information on just about any topic of interest. So, when we decide to embark on a change in lifestyle, we do our homework. Such research is commendable, but it can soon result in a mountain of expert opinions, confusion and a potential loss of resolve. Believe me, I know! I've been there myself.

Like many of you, I read everything I can get my hands on about health—not just science journals and textbooks, but also ads for health products, popular magazines and articles on the Web. Again, much of what I read seems to step over many fundamental concepts of biochemistry that have been accepted by scientists for the better part of the last century. This prevailing oversight may be a result of the same problem I faced when I tried to learn how to apply what I had learned about biochemistry and physiology in order to better my own health. I found that these basic concepts had not yet been translated into practical guidelines for living. It also seems, for the most part, that they have not been taught to parents, teachers, children or even to medical doctors and pharmacists. Where can we find the reliable guidelines we so desperately need?

It's only those people who have studied nutrition who seem to have some understanding of these basics. I say this because, in my experience, it is nutritionists (or health professionals who have taken on nutrition as an additional field of interest) who have written the best books and articles that I've read on the topic of health. I'm thinking of authors such as Jean Carper, Ann Louise Gittleman, Carol Simontacchi, and Lillian Grant. Chiropractors and naturopaths, who prescribe alternatives to pharmaceutical therapies, should also be commended for their advocacy of good nutrition and holistic healthcare.

Historically, medical schools have offered very little in the way of training around nutrition. A 1998 survey showed that only 26% of accredited medical schools had a required nutrition course. A more recent survey points to an increased awareness of this shortcoming, as medical schools are now requiring more hours of nutrition education (Torti, et al., 2001). Thus, we can hope that future medical school graduates will be more prepared to answer the growing public demand for professional advice on nutrition.

I believe that past ignorance of the fundamental concepts of biochemistry and physiology is responsible for the grim statistics we see in the occurrence of degenerative diseases, and also contributes to the lack of agreement or clear insight about what can be done to address this growing concern. One clear consequence of this ignorance is seen in how professional athletes deal with their health. For example, our culture invests heavily in professional sports—time, energy and big bucks—and fans and backers expect results. For this reason, many athletes have considered the use of steroids, metabolic boosters or various supplements in order to enhance their performance. Ironically, at the same time they have been ignoring the basic needs of their body chemistry. Or is it that athletes were never educated about these basic needs to begin with? Unfortunately, the sum of what many athletes know is from the pages of popular magazines and hard sell advertising brochures. It's amazing to me how these athletes seem to succeed in spite of their eating habits and training routines; I've seen elite athletes, after a race, reaching for a soft drink and a candy bar. These athletes are a testament to how much abuse a young body can tolerate. Growing old gracefully requires us to treat the body with more reverence.

Not only are the basics being overlooked, but also when new research is presented, it often gets reported to the public in such a way as to skew the fundamental concepts. For instance, one of the many prime-time ads for pharmaceuticals recently caught my eye; a drug company was describing how they would be able to take advantage of the findings of the Human Genome Project in the not-so-distant future by providing people with genetic ID cards. According to the ad, a physician would be able to use one of these cards to identify troublesome genes in a patient and then be able to prescribe pills that could prevent the onset of diseases, such as cancer. That sounds good. But, if we examine this claim in light of the fundamental concepts of biochemistry and physiology, the ad is very misleading to the public. First of all, it ignores the long-known fact that genetics does not determine everything—environment plays a role as well. Second, a pill to prevent cancer is a bit of a stretch (for reasons that will become clear later in this book). Third, and perhaps most disturbing, with so many companies claiming patents on various human genes (which, by the way, sounds absurd to me), the ad verges on propaganda: "Hey, let us keep patenting these genes, because we have your best interests at heart." In reality, genetic profiling may someday threaten our right to receive jobs or health insurance. In the future, companies may choose to add a genetic blueprint to their selection criteria—right after the mandatory drug test.

Obviously, some of these concerns relate to the not-so-distant future; but the general public's lack of understanding about the fundamentals of biochemistry has already contributed to an often unwarranted dependence on pharmaceuticals and, hence, to the profits of pharmaceutical suppliers. It has a far-reaching consequence in helping to determine the amount and allocation of monies for general research. Fundraising events aimed at raising money to cure a specific disease have been a particular source of personal frustration. For instance, I've gone to fund-raisers for breast cancer and been torn between the cause itself and the purpose for which the money was being solicited. I'm heartbroken when I hear cancer survivors or any ill person describe what it's like, living with the disease and the treatments; but when the spokesperson begins to explain where the money might be going, I'm always left with the feeling that much of it will be wasted. Let me explain. I believe that the majority of the funds raised should not be spent on looking for putative cures, as they have been spent historically. With any disease that we hope to cure, it's imperative that our major emphasis be on educating people. Lifestyle changes are important not only for prevention of the disease to begin with, but also for recovery and protection against recurrence.

When you boil it down to the basics, the principles for staying healthy or reviving health are really very simple;

hopefully, you will agree with me after you've read this book. I don't claim to have all the answers, and new dilemmas arise daily. In fact, much of the delay between the conceiving and writing of this book has had to do with the fact that I didn't want to advocate possibilities, or even probabilities, that might be disproved in the days ahead. Such is the nature of science, however, that no one has ever written a book that marked progress or made a difference in the world without some parts of it being wrong. Even so, it's still important to engage in the process of putting forward new ideas and new ways of thinking. By the way, I certainly don't mean to give the impression that all of these provocative new ideas originated with me. I've made a serious effort to cite my sources whenever possible. Of course, there are also those colleagues who have mentioned an idea to me in an elevator at a conference, or friends who have led me to a new realization while we were chatting on the phone. There is no way to thank the many people who have inspired me to keep searching for answers. There are still so many mysteries, so many health practices, that I don't yet understand; but, as a scientist, I can't merely dismiss them. Some medical professionals may choose to say "Nonsense!" to alternative practices; but, in science, not understanding something can never be grounds for dismissing it. Furthermore, what purpose can be served by quarreling over various approaches to health and healing: a naturopath and a medical doctor need not be on guard against each other; after all, in the end, they're both interested in the same result. It seems to me that we have much more to learn from one another than to dispute over.

Early memories of small white sugar pills and clear liquids

that tasted slightly different from plain old water, remind me to be humble, and realize that what I think I understand about modern science and medicine is at best a fraction of the whole picture. What I'm describing are the homeopathic remedies given to me by my grandfather while I was growing up in Kolkata (formerly Calcutta), India. Homeopathic remedies are counter-intuitive for most people and certainly not predicted by the laws of chemistry. The word "homeopathy" means "similar suffering"; and the Law of Similars, on which homeopathy is based, says that what a substance can cause, it can also cure. Perhaps an analogy will help to illustrate how the Law of Similars works. If you were troubled by a particular noise and wanted to drown it out, you would not use a beam of light, but rather you might reproduce that noise and then modulate the phase, so that the waves of noise could cancel each other out. Or consider waves in the ocean. When one wave is coming in and another is going back out, where they meet, you suddenly see the waves disappear. They have, as with the waves of sound in the ocean of air, cancelled each other out. Now, when Samuel Hahnemann, the founder of the formal system of homeopathy, first started using the Law of Similars, he found that his patients could be aggravated by a crude dose of a treatment to the point of their lives being in danger. Diluting the treatment, he knew, would render it too weak to be effective. Somehow, he came upon the idea of "succession," which required a specific amount of vigorous shaking at each stage of dilution. Using this concept, he could eventually have a dilution where there was no material particle of the original substance left. As such, these diluted solutions did not cause any adverse effects and yet, they still retained the ability to remedy the illness. Furthermore, he found that each stage of dilution and succession renders a more potent remedy (Wells, 1993). The implication is that the water in which the active chemical is suspended retains a memory of the molecule as a result of the vigorous shaking.

Do I believe this and do I ask you to believe this? I can only tell you that my world as a young girl in Kolkata was quite different from the one in the United States where I would eventually train in the philosophies of modern science. During my tenure as a graduate student at Stanford, I remember that there was a very controversial article published in a leading scientific journal, *Nature*, on the possibility of homeopathic principles being validated by modern experimentation (Davenas, et al., 1988). It raised quite a few eyebrows to say the least. This article suggested that diluting a chemical agent to the order of one part per 10^{120} (that is, 1 with one hundred and twenty 0's after it) still allows that chemical's properties to be retained. Since there would be no original chemical left at that dilution, the implication was that this was possibly due to water having a "memory" of that chemical, which could manifest itself in cycles of dilution and vigorous shaking. This method, as I explained earlier, is called "succession" in homeopathy.

For me, it was an extraordinary moment in science. I thought that my two worlds were destined to collide, and that I would finally understand homeopathy. It would have been one thing if the experiments had been based on previously verified facts—for instance, if it had already been proven that water could take on a molecular configuration that had the ability to heal an illness. It would have helped if an independent party could have repeated the experiments. It was not as convincing because the results could be explained by other models besides the homeopathic model. But none of these criteria were met and so the journal duly dismissed the original article (Maddox, et al., 1988).

While homeopathy has not met the standards of modern science, it has influenced my personal life—even if only at the level of a powerful placebo. Interestingly, it wasn't until my parents and I came down with chicken pox as adults living in the United States that I fully realized how much homeopathy had shaped my family's life in India. When I asked my mom why we had not gotten chicken pox as children in Kolkata, she told me that her father had always given everyone in the house a homeopathic remedy to fight chicken pox; but when my grandfather passed away, our regular homeopathic treatments ceased with him. When we later moved to the United States, we didn't think to worry about being exposed to chickenpox as adults. We took no precautions, and thus defenseless against chicken pox, eventually, we got it. That's the story anyway.

Moving to the United States had other consequences for my family's health. For one, my parents regularly experienced the stress and financial pressure of being first generation immigrants. My father was a civil engineer, and the 1970s were not good years for this profession. One by one, his colleagues were being laid off from work. He was feeling the strain of adjusting to a new country, with a wife and two children to feed and a mortgage to pay. To make matters worse for his health, he smoked. But even with all these strikes against him, my father still had an amazing ability to convince everyone who knew him that he was healthy and happy.

When we woke up on weekends, my younger brother and I couldn't wait to run into our parents' bedroom and jump up and down on their bed. Meanwhile, my father would lay there and groan to my mom in the kitchen for *cha*, which is Bengali for "tea." One such morning, his groans sounded alarmingly different. He was having a massive myocardial infarction—a heart attack. Within 15 minutes he was rushed to a state-of-the-art cardiovascular wing of a large hospital, which just happened to be right in the town where we lived. That fact alone may have saved his life then. As it turned out, he was one of the first in a long line of his Indian, first generation male friends to have heart problems. At that time, I was only 12 years of age, but old enough to take note of what smoking and stress could do. And so it was that both my brother and I made one of those earnest vows that children make—we pledged to become doctors and save the world from heart attacks.

Alas, two years later, I found myself hating 9th grade biology. During the rest of my time in high school, I excelled in math and physics instead. It was not until after I graduated from Cornell University with a Bachelors degree in Electrical Engineering that I began to find biology interesting. I was encouraged by a professor at Stanford University, while I was interviewing for graduate schools, to pursue a whole different line of study—cellular physiology and bio-chemistry. I was intrigued by how cells carried electrochemical signals and how biological neural networks were even more intricate than the artificial intelligence algorithms I had studied in engineering school. I began my graduate studies at Stanford Medical School, hurrying to make up for my lack of undergraduate training in biology; but my engineering background was to come in very handy in the lab, helping me set up experiments that used some of the latest techniques in biophysics.

While I toiled in basic research, something was happening to my own body. I was only 21 years old when I entered graduate school, but I had started to age rapidly. No one would ever have guessed by looking at me. Besides, I was so active. I was swimming in a wonderful pool at Stanford where they train their Olympic-level athletes. I was playing ultimate Frisbee several times a week. I commuted to the lab on my bicycle, riding over 10 miles a day. During the winter, I was skiing at Lake Tahoe; and during the rest of the year, I was hiking, climbing and kayaking. I would also run in the foothills around the campus. It was on one such run that an old injury from bodysurfing during my teens came back to haunt me. In the middle of my run, I started to experience an excruciating pain in my neck. It took all the energy I had to get myself back to the campus. This was the beginning of chronic back spasms that were to become more and more frequent with time. The pain was so bad during one siege that I was given morphine and stayed in bed for a whole week. X-rays showed nothing. Doctors could only advise me to start curtailing my active lifestyle. I took enough ibuprofen, as suggested by my doctor for the pain, to give myself an ulcer. I was also drinking about 5 cups of coffee a day and not sleeping well at night.

Five years later, as I was starting post-graduate research, I was seeing a physical therapist several times a week to manage the pain I was feeling in my neck from hovering over a microscope all day. Yet, if you had asked me then whether I was healthy or not, I would probably have said "Other than my neck, I'm really in pretty good shape." Maybe I was in denial, but there was no doctor telling me anything different. After all, my blood pressure was low; my cholesterol was low; my heartbeat was low; my weight was average; I was very strong; and, I was still very active in between back spasm episodes.

Two years later, at age 28, I had curtailed my activity enough that I started to gain a little weight; and that's what finally motivated me to read about health and nutrition. I became fascinated with juicing and the possibility that plant enzymes and coenzymes could have tremendous health benefits. The literature on juicing was not scientific at all. From my understanding, before scientists had discovered a way to isolate enzymes without losing their innate biological activity, they had thought that there was some "life force" that people would never really be able to understand which existed in food and other living things. The "life force" idea still prevailed in the books that I was reading on juicing; these books talked about the power of "live" juices, which I gathered meant that heat had not destroyed most of the nutritional and enzymatic value as it does in cooked vegetables.

On the other hand, there were plenty of scientific studies on the power of vegetables and fruits. Although it was hard for me to comprehend juicing broccoli or cranberries, I began juicing the more palatable veggies and fruits, like apples and carrots, and it did increase my overall energy level. Working 10-14 hours in the lab, usually six to seven days a week, I certainly appreciated the energy boost. Then, I was introduced to a new supplement on the market called Juice Plus+® that was essentially the "live" juices from 17 veggies and fruits that had been lyophilized—that is, dehydrated in a vacuum in the presence of liquid nitrogen so as to retain biological activity even after dehydration. I had one of those "AHA!!" moments. I kicked myself for not thinking of that idea myself, but promptly ordered some. I had never been able to keep a vitamin pill down, so I was intrigued by the concept of food concentrates.

After taking this supplement twice a day for six weeks, my physical therapist asked me if I was doing something different. My neck had begun to loosen up. It seems to be human nature that we concentrate less on the things that are going well, but her words made me take notice of other improvements. I was naturally drinking less coffee, because I was not feeling that afternoon lull. I was sleeping better at night; my clothes were looser on me; and, the list goes on. So I got curious and went back to the library. I read some 200 abstracts and a few dozen papers on vegetables and fruits and became convinced that eating more vegetables and fruits, especially uncooked, was a critical step for my health.

Now some people are wired in such a way that when they find out something good, they just have to tell others. I'm definitely one of those people. So I started telling everyone. Some people were skeptical. They argued that what I was experiencing was a placebo effect; although later I'll share some research that shows this was not purely placebo.

One of my biochemist friends actually said, "Oh, come on, we're engineered to draw sustenance from Twinkies® if we need to." I realized that if a biochemist could dismiss the long-term cost of drawing sustenance from Twinkies® (and it is highly questionable whether we are engineered for even short-term gain from Twinkies®), then what about the average person? The irony is that I, myself, had been funded by the American Cancer Society, the National Institutes of Health, and the Alzheimer's Society to study how cells work and to determine the possible causes of diseases like cancer and Alzheimer's. Even so, I knew very little about how to take care of my own health.

I think that it takes a lot of energy and perseverance to wade through the sea of information that we're bombarded with today. Nevertheless, it is critical for our health that we make sense of what is important, and then apply it, if we want our lives to work. In my attempts to explain to others about this new path I was traveling down, I found holes in my knowledge base, made apparent by the fact that I couldn't always answer people's questions. So I began to read more; concurrently, I opened my mind to other methods of healing. For instance, people had recommended chiropractors to me before. "Are you kidding?" I would say. I was scared to death of letting someone "crack" my neck. Chiropractic care did not fit into the medical and scientific world in which I lived at that point in my life, and I was happy to be scared of it. But with some urging from friends who'd had positive results with chiropractic care, I was willing to take another look. And pretty soon, I was seeing a chiropractor. For the first time, someone was taking X-rays of my neck and pointing out what was wrong, instead of parroting what

I had been hearing for years prior to this, which was, "We don't see any problems." The problems that the X-rays showed as explained by the chiropractor made sense to me, and I began to respect and appreciate this method of treatment. Since I had already been to reputable sports medicine clinics and seen several orthopedists who had offered no hope for my situation, I appreciated my chiropractor's saying that I was young enough that the problem was probably reversible. Suddenly, the fog that had descended when I thought that I would have to live with horrible back spasms for the rest of my life was starting to lift. It's not that I'm endorsing chiropractic care over, say, orthopedic care; but on the road to healing, finding a competent professional with the right attitude has proven to be just as beneficial to me as the method of treatment. Perhaps there are chiropractors who would have been less effective or perhaps I didn't talk to the right orthopedist. My point is that in order for my body to heal, I had to first reject the notion that it couldn't heal. Then I had to keep searching for solutions and approach the problem from every possible angle, not just nutrition alone, stress management alone, or exercise alone.

As my body began to heal and my medicine cabinet emptied out, I started to work with other people on their health. My motivation was to help others with the monumental task of sifting through all of the information that's available; I wanted to come up with easy and workable guidelines for creating health and vitality. I also wanted to reach as many people as possible, as quickly as possible. I found an interesting opportunity to make audiotapes of my lectures and reach a sizeable audience through the company that markets Juice Plus+®—NSA, Inc. (Please read *To My*

Readers on page vii at the front of this book.) Since I was already recommending their food concentrate product, I had a natural forum for teaching people the basics of how the body works. I was amazed that my talks inspired people to change their daily habits. All they'd needed was someone to treat them like intelligent human beings, and to finally explain to them the fundamental principles that we'll talk about in this book. My one-on-one counseling was very straightforward. I wouldn't hold people's hands. I would tell people to listen to my tape, over and over again if need be, and start to make the lifestyle changes I suggested. To this day, I'm surprised at how many people shower me with cards, gifts and heartfelt compliments on how I've turned their lives around. According to them, all they had to do was to attend a lecture or listen to a tape and then heed the advice. My congratulations to those who have listened and have heard, to those who choose health every day of their lives. In turn, I also wish to thank all those who requested that I write this book; by encouraging you to move beyond your self-imposed barriers, I've found the inspiration to continue to travel there myself. This book, then, is for you.

In these pages, my goal is to provide a comprehensive overview of the concepts you will need to know in order to restore or maintain health. I hope to instill in you a level of confidence and understanding of these concepts that will allow you to apply them in your daily life; and, as a result, to experience a sense of more abundant health. These are concepts that are scientifically sound. These are methods that work. Then, there are methods that seem to work, but don't fit the scientific mold; I'll also discuss my views on many of these methods throughout the book. For now, let me say that I am not writing this book as a scientist, surveying the land of research related to health. Rather, I am writing this book as a human being with a background in science, sorting through information, raising important questions, looking for answers, and distinguishing methods that either already have scientific merit, or make sense based on known facts, but perhaps haven't been fully proven yet.

First, we'll look at the state of health in our society today. I call this our "Default Health Program." We'll look at how our health is impacted by the use of pharmaceuticals, the effects of our environment and the effects of our lifestyle. Then, we'll consider what it is to break free of the Default Health Program and what longevity really means. In order to obtain our goal of longevity, three important factors cannot be overlooked: *nutrition, stress physiology* and *exercise physiology.* This book will help you become well-grounded in the fundamental principles of these three areas. Every time a new book or fad comes along, you won't get confused, then deterred and ultimately frustrated. You'll have the knowledge and confidence to keep traveling down your own road to longevity.

2

The Default Health Program

It wasn't until I was 28 years old and grappling with intense pain and weight gain that I was finally willing to take full responsibility for my health. What I'd been experiencing slowly over time was the downward spiral of health that I now call "the Default Health Program." Even today, unless I'm watchful, I know that I can slip back into that program. Our experience of the Default Health Program goes something like this: we may say that we want to make health a priority, but we don't do that. We eat whatever is readily available or what's easy to buy or heat up. Maybe we exercise and maybe we don't. We allow the daily stresses of career and family to get the best of us. When we get a headache, we swallow some aspirin or rush to buy that new "wonder drug" we heard about on TV. Sometimes we can't sleep at night, so we try an herbal tea as a home remedy. Eventually, this casual approach to our health catches up with us. We get so sick that we end up going to a clinic, where we get a diagnosis. With prescription in hand, we go to the pharmacy, pick up a drug, and start taking it without paying much attention the list of side effects and contraindications. What does "contraindication" mean anyway? Sometimes we get really preoccupied with the diagnosis and start our own research project to find out more about what's happened to us. Then all of our focus is on what went wrong. Managing and treating what's wrong with us is what we call healthcare. Actually, it's sick care. That is, we only seem to care when we are sick!

When insurance companies choose to pay for a medical bill, they usually pay for sick care, but seldom pay for wellness care or prevention. We should realize that this choice is based on simple economics. In the past, the average time that an employee remained with a company was 25 years or more. Today, an employee is projected to change jobs an average of 10 times over a 45-year working period; thus, an employer has no financial interest in investing in what a person's health will be 10 years from now. If an employee gets sick and misses work, it only makes financial sense for an employer to pay the least amount of money that will manage the current symptoms and get that employee back on the job.

Likewise, pharmaceutical companies have to concentrate on the bottom line. So, why would they invest research and development (R&D) dollars on a one time cure, when they can have people take a maintenance drug that wards off symptoms, for as long as possible? From their point of view, this is just good business. When you and I practice prevention, we become part of a growing financial threat to pharmaceutical companies. When you're willing to make some significant changes in your Default Health Program, you and your doctor may find that you are able to reduce or, eventually, to eliminate your need for prescription drugs. You will also have lessened your risk of suffering from any side effects associated with those drugs. You will have begun to break out of the downward spiral. If you don't stop or back off from this process of breaking free, and are willing to experience the symptoms that your body is giving you, you can become more aware of what your body needs. As you move from treating symptoms to truly healing your body, your need for pharmaceuticals should logically diminish. Now, I'm not saying that you should stop taking your meds. That may or may not be appropriate for you, as we'll discuss in the next chapter. My point here is that from a financial perspective, drug companies have little interest in your wellness. They are counting on you to stay focussed on your illness. They profit by helping you to manage your symptoms. On the other hand, nutritional supplementation companies and your local grocer want you to practice prevention; and they, not unlike the drug companies, also want you to take their products for the rest of your life. The difference is that they profit by having you live a long life that is focussed on wellness.

We have the power to make conscious, informed choices about how, where and when we will spend money on our health. *We can invest in our wellness or subsidize our illness.* For me, it wasn't until I started to hurt that I was finally able to accept responsibility for my own health. It hadn't occurred to me that chiropractic care, massage, yoga, and something as simple as eating better could help prevent something like back spasms. Since I had originally hurt my back as a teenager, I thought that my back spasms were merely the consequence of continually tweaking an injured muscle that hadn't had enough time to heal properly. I would never have imagined that my diet, hectic lifestyle and lack of appropriate exercise were all contributing to the escalation of the original back injury. Eventually, I found myself buying ibuprofen in bulk, and seeing a physical therapist several times a week in order to try to manage the pain. I thought that taking painkillers was a code of honor for active people. Practicing preventative medicine was not a part of my daily agenda. Instead, I had been unknowingly participating in my own Default Health Program.

To further illustrate what I mean by the Default Health Program, let's think about the way computers operate. Computers, as you may already know, come with basic programs already installed. For instance, there's a default setting for the background color of your screen, which will run unless you change it. There are many examples of default programming in our daily lives as well. We often celebrate holidays in the same particular ways our families have always celebrated them. These default programs become the norm, and it usually takes some outside force to change them. Similarly, each of us has a default program that runs us. Unfortunately, this default program is not always a well-designed and useful program that guides us toward longevity; rather, it often runs us into the ground.

As you might imagine, the default program thrives on the hectic lifestyle that's prevalent in our society today. Most of our lives consist of too much to do and not enough time. As we dash through the day, the widespread availability of prepared foods and junk food makes it easy for us to eat on the run. We have "the need for speed," and today's modern conveniences, such as automobiles, escalators, and "people movers" in airports, make it easier for us to avoid exercise, and get there faster. Our jobs may be sedentary, our heads spinning with financial worries, but when our bodies start to fall apart, we have a cornucopia of pharmaceuticals to help us perpetuate the Default Health Program.

As shown in the following diagram, the Default Health Program looks from the perspective of the end result—the Effect. That is to say, sick care (or healthcare, as we have come to call it) provides treatments that are disease-specific.

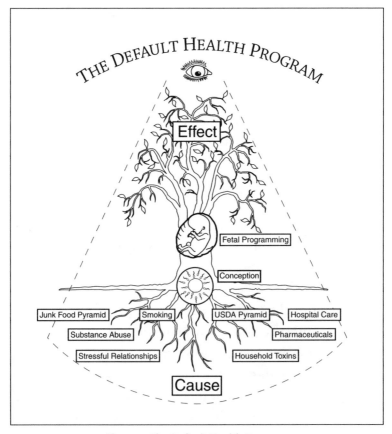

Figure 1. The Default Health Program

But people don't have singular diseases; they have multiple diseases that get independently diagnosed over time. Sick care is looking from the perspective of the barren branches of the tree, wondering why there is no fruit; meanwhile, the roots, the Cause, are being fed the various aspects of the Default Health Program. In the course of this book, we'll discuss each of these aspects and how it contributes to ill health; but, even now, I think that you can begin to see that healthcare needs to change its perspective—from Effect to Cause. We need to focus on what is working in the body and take care of this part. In order to maintain and regain our health, we need to feed the roots of the tree with aspects that promote health, that are based in prevention. This means that, if we want to live life to its fullest potential, if we want the tree to bear fruit, we must do our best to protect the DNA that we were born with from damage and mutations.

Think about it this way: whether you are already suffering from a disease or whether you were born with a genetic predisposition for a particular disease, you still want to increase your odds by practicing prevention. Since most of us can assume that our DNA at conception was healthy, then the road to longevity is about protecting this DNA as best we can from the dangers of modern living.

You probably noticed the simple dictionary definition of "longevity" at the beginning of this book; but in order to really understand what is meant by "longevity," it's important to understand that we were not born with a predetermined DNA program for aging, nor is aging a disease. That is, there isn't a DNA message saying, "Hey, it's time to give this guy heart disease or arthritis. Let's throw in a little osteoporosis while we're at it." Aging doesn't have to include diseases, such as stroke, cancer and heart disease; yet most of research is focused on finding cures for these diseases, since statistics would lead us to believe that they are inevitable.

Now you may have heard on the news that some people really *are* programmed to live longer lives. Yes, it's true that some of us may possess genes that help us age more gracefully; by studying siblings that all seem to live a long and healthy life, researchers have recently shown the location of what seem to be longevity genes that allow people to live a healthy life beyond 100 years of age (Puca et al., 2001). Be that as it may, I'm here to tell you that there's plenty of evidence to support the notion that the rest of us can also increase our odds of achieving longevity—if we'll just start making the best of the genes that we've been dealt.

This book is generally a discussion of why and how diseases are preventable; but for now, let's consider what it would mean for us, as a society, if we were able to find these promised cures. It might surprise you to learn that even if we were able to cure heart disease, stroke and cancer this would only increase our average life expectancy by perhaps 15 years (Hayflick, 2000). In addition, such cures wouldn't necessarily provide us with more insight into why we age or how to achieve longevity. There is currently no reason to believe that such cures will be found; however, this fact has done nothing to stanch the flow of propaganda about miracle cures. Let's say that these imagined cures actually existed and we were fortunate enough to ultimately discover them, there is no guarantee that a whole new set of diseases would not emerge down the road.

Aging is usually defined as "the progressive loss of function accompanied by decreasing fertility and increasing mortality with advancing age" (Kirkwood and Austad, 2000). In other words, as we age, we lose our ability to reproduce, our senses diminish and our chances of dying go up. So what's the big deal? Who didn't know that? Well, the problem is that people are living longer today; and, as a result, we are experiencing firsthand all the many ways in which it's possible to lose facility and function. I will grant that modern medicine has been successful at trying to make this process less painful; but why should we expect that it has to be this way to begin with? Besides, less pain does not necessarily equal less suffering. There are many other costs to disease: worried family members, less productivity, low self-esteem and high medical bills. The real challenge is not just to live longer, but also to age gracefully. This means we have to change our focus from merely trying to ease the pain of degenerative disease; instead, we need to focus on all of the possible ways that we can stay well.

The alternative is to live a fairly long life—certainly longer than cave dwellers lived—but to become dependent on drugs, artificial machinery and other people for assisted living. Aside from the work being done in the area of infectious diseases, most of current research and medicine is aimed towards getting better and better at taking care of sick people as they age. I assert that this approach misses the mark. If we are to choose an ideal to strive for, should it be merely to ease the pain of those who are suffering from disease? Or should it be to prevent disease in the first place? It's not enough to assist people in living a longer life, without the promise of a quality of life—right to the very end. My wish for you is that when it is your time to go, you can die peacefully in your sleep—of old age.

When I finally realized this extremely important concept, it forever altered the way I wanted to participate in research. I could no longer justify writing research grant proposals to study various disease processes. As a biochemist, I realized that most of the research related to disease is focused on what, in the final analysis, is an inevitable outcome of the body's not having been taken good care of in the first place.

Think of it like this: the way in which society goes about trying to understand and cure a disease can be compared to the study of sociopathic behavior. When we, as a society, spend all of our time and resources trying to determine what random childhood event or sequence of events might have caused a person to become a sociopath, we are ignoring the possibility of prevention. By spending adequate resources on trying to raise today's children with love, a sense of security, and proper nutrition (see *Chapter Seven*), we have an opportunity to address the root cause, rather than commenting on the effect. While our current approach may provide some insight into what causes disease or what sets off a sociopath, that information doesn't serve us unless we utilize it to prevent such disasters. I assert that we have enough information about how to raise healthy, functioning members of society, but that this information is not making a difference. We need to take action now. Just as we should focus more on how today's children are being raised if we want to build a better society for the future, we need also to focus on the prevention of diseases if we want a long and healthy life for every member of that society.

In today's society, old people have multiple pathologies, and since we don't do autopsies on each and every individual who dies, we rarely know the true cause of death. What we do know about aging is that some time after we have attained a fixed adult size, and we have passed our reproductive years, the ability to maintain the fidelity of genes and cells starts to diminish. Yet, it is intriguing to look at certain species that do not reach a fixed adult size, such as some turtles, many sport and cold-water deep-sea fish, some amphibians and the American lobster, and recognize that these animals may not age at all. In our current understanding, infectious disease, predation and accidents seem to be the only causes that keep them from being immortal (Ibid., p. 267). Rather than focusing our efforts on the end point of disease, perhaps it would be more productive to spend our time and money studying these animals in order to determine why they don't seem to age in the first place.

Unfortunately, health care's fixation on Effect rather than Cause has resulted in a preponderance of research on age-related disease (the field of geriatric medicine) rather than on why or how we age (biogerontology). This, in turn, has had many socio-political and economic consequences. For instance, *more than half* the budget of the U.S. National Institute on Aging is spent on research for Alzheimer's disease, even though the likelihood of dying from Alzheimer's disease is only 0.7%, and a cure would only increase the average life expectancy by perhaps 19 days (Ibid., p. 267).

That is to say, yes, I do agree that Alzheimer's disease is a tragic disease to live with. This common sentiment seems to justify the large proportion of funds that the U.S. National Institute on Aging allocates towards finding a cure. But, the cure is so unlikely that this spending may not only be unwarranted, but also, perhaps, irrational. If, on the other hand, that money were spent mostly on the *prevention* of Alzheimer's disease, then that would have the potential of increasing the quality of life for everyone. Now, I understand that if someone in your family were to suffer from Alzheimer's and eventually to pass away, you might be moved to request that donations be made to Alzheimer's research, in lieu of flowers. Yet, if we lived in a world where an autopsy were performed, as a matter of course, on every person who died, you might be told that your loved one had also had a failing heart and a diseased liver. My point is that the very idea that we can ever diagnose a single disease or even a single cause of death may be a fallacy. We have a healthcare system based on the end point of disease, when that very end point can never be stated with absolute certainty.

Should we spend more time and money looking for that elusive end point? So far, the search hasn't significantly reduced human suffering. The problem stems from the fact that a plethora of lifestyle and environmental factors can damage our DNA, which in turn can cause enzymatic pathways to arbitrarily go astray, resulting in disease. Think of it this way: we get sick because our genes have somehow taken a wrong turn. Then we try to discover where and how that turn was made instead of trying to stay on the right path in the first place. As you can imagine, it's been a slow and tedious task to study disease from this end; and, ironically, even when scientists have succeeded in explaining the arbitrary disease pathway, it hasn't made it any easier to get things back on the right track. After so much time and so much money, we still haven't really found cures for the most prevalent diseases that plague us today—heart disease, stroke and cancer. And, as I mentioned earlier, even if we did find cures for all three of these diseases, experts predict that it would only increase life expectancy by 15 years (Ibid., p. 267; Anderson, 1999). Of course, 15 years is 15 years! But evidence suggests that if we were to invest our time and money in prevention, it might yield higher dividends.

Later on, we'll talk about some of the factors that can damage or mutate the DNA that we were born with, such as junk food, stress and exercise; but first, let's look at the final component of our Default Health Program—pharmaceuticals. In order to break free of this vicious cycle, it's important to recognize where such a program can lead us. Do we really want to spend our lives as diseased and drug-dependent human beings? If we look at centenarians—people who live to be over 100 years of age—they generally aren't pill-popping machines. The road to longevity does not have to include pharmaceuticals.

3

Drug-Free America

I once offended someone when I showed the following cartoon in a lecture, because her son had ADHD and she felt that I wasn't sympathizing with her. My purpose in sharing this cartoon would never be to judge people. There are obviously many instances in which a disease has progressed to the point where strenuous intervention is necessary; in

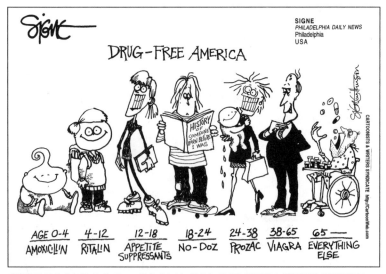

©SIGNE *Philadelphia Daily News*, Philadelphia, U.S.A. CARTOONISTS & WRITERS SYNDICATE, http://CartoonWeb.com

such cases, pharmaceuticals can often prolong life or, at the very least, make an illness more bearable. There are some medications, however, that could be avoided, or gradually replaced, by looking to the root cause of the body's complaint and making the appropriate lifestyle changes. Pharmaceuticals should not be used in every instance, as a matter of course, simply because they're available to us.

I have elected to use the cartoon because it graphically illustrates our growing dependence on drugs and because it practically screams the question: "Do we overuse pharmaceuticals?" Furthermore, it suggests the follow-up question: "Wouldn't it be worth our while to explore alternatives to pharmaceuticals?"

I ask these two questions of everyone, even the president or CEO of a pharmaceutical company, who may be immensely wealthy from drug patents. These questions and the discussion they elicit are meant to alert us to the current state of healthcare in America. We all, individually and as a society, have contributed to the current dilemmas facing our healthcare system. Worrying about who is ultimately responsible is neither useful nor practical. And, quite frankly, we don't have the time. Instead, we all need to wake up to the fact that habitually medicating the body has grave consequences—for each of us, for our families and for our society in general.

While we can all take some personal responsibility in the matter, we certainly can't let pharmaceutical companies completely off the hook. Please understand that I'm not taking issue with capitalism. My husband and I are entrepreneurs ourselves. But, in the wise words of Mahatma Gandhi, "Science without humanity and commerce without morality" are two of the seven deadly sins.[1] Pharmaceutical companies spent half a billion dollars on advertising in the year 2000 (Avila, 2001). Why? Because it works: people now ask their doctors for expensive, state-of-the-art medications by name. Americans spent $111.1 billion on outpatient prescription drugs in 1999. In the year 2000 alone, that figure rose by 18.8% to $131.9 billion. The bulk of this growth was attributable to a small number of categories of drugs, where new, expensive brand names brought in more sales. It's important to note that the average cost of most drugs has gone down, as long as you stay away from the top four brand names. For instance, if you were looking for a generic antidepressant, the average price for a prescription was $45.11 in 2000, as compared to $48.82 in 1998. But if you wanted one of the comparable brand names, it would have cost you a great deal more: Celexa was priced at $69.05; Paxil, at $78.62; and Wellbutrin, at $85.88 in 2000.

The average cost of generic oral antidiabetics was $27.27

Medication	1998	2000
Generic Antidepressants	$48.82	$45.11
Celexa		69.05
Paxil		78.62
Wellbutrin		85.88
Generic Oral Antidiabetics	$34.18	$27.27
Avancia		116.27
Actos		137.57

Figure 2. Comparing Prices of "Designer" and Generic Drugs

[1] In case you find yourself curious about what Gandhi considered to be the other five sins, they are: wealth without work, pleasure without conscience, knowledge without character, worship without sacrifice, and politics without principle.

in 2000, down from $34.18 in 1998. Again, if you preferred
brand names, Avandia was $116.27 and Actos was $137.57
in 2000. Similar comparisons can be made for antiulcer
drugs, cholesterol reducers, arthritis drugs, antibiotics,
painkillers, HIV/AIDS treatments and respiratory steroids
(NIH report, 2001). Pharmaceutical companies will argue
that these newer brand-name/"designer" drugs are more
effective. Well, I should hope so at these prices! But, can we
afford these runaway prices as a society? And why is it that
Europeans and Asians pay a lot less for drugs than we do in
the United States?

According to an article in *The Seattle Times* newspaper,
lawmakers in the state of Washington are "facing the
grimmest budget outlook in nearly a decade, largely
because medical spending for public employees, prisoners,
the poor and others is expected to grow by more than
$1 billion over the next two years" (Thomas, 2001). State
capitals across the nation are facing this type of fiscal
challenge. Moreover, what is it costing us as individuals,
especially considering that many of the conditions being
treated might have been preventable in the first place?

Much of the training and daily practice of medical professionals involves dispensing pharmaceuticals; and when I
suggest that we might be overusing pharmaceuticals, I
know that I run the risk of alienating a large segment of the
medical community. I would like to say, especially to them,
that I don't think that physicians went to school with the
dream of dispensing pharmaceuticals all day long. The
dream is to help people. Yet, in trying to deal with large
numbers of people who are overworked, overstressed,

undernourished and suffering, physicians rarely have the time they would like to devote to individual counseling. Likewise, often patients themselves are unwilling or unable to invest the time to work toward a cure, but instead will settle for a "quick fix." The patient will ask, "Can you give me a pill or something? I can't miss any more days at work." Influenced by powerful advertising in the media, patients are even requesting medications by name. In this climate, dispensing pharmaceuticals becomes the necessary norm; many physicians have expressed their frustration that the traditional role of the healer has been reduced to that of a salesperson for pharmaceutical companies (Bland, 2001).

How did we become a society so dependent on pharmaceuticals? There are other cultures where people live to a ripe old age without ever taking over-the-counter or prescription medicines. Let's consider two important aspects of this question:

- Are pharmaceuticals effective in the treatment of disease?
- Are there viable alternatives to pharmaceuticals?

This chapter is, for the most part, an inquiry into the effectiveness of drugs, while the remainder of the book will explore the alternatives. I'll do my best to supply you with the information you'll need in order to make informed choices. In the end, it's up to each of you to determine what the answers are.

To assist us in our search for answers, let's take a brief look at the two major philosophies of medicine and healing, as they are being practiced or applied in the world today.

We'll look first at Vitalism, also known as Empiricism. Homeopathy is based on the philosophy of Vitalism, which is shared by naturopathic doctors and other holistic practitioners. It states that the whole body is greater than the sum of its parts, and considers the synergistic effects of the parts on the whole. According to Vitalism, it isn't possible to treat one part without affecting the whole. For example, if you came down with a fever and went to see a homeopathic doctor, he or she wouldn't just treat the fever. Rather, you and the doctor would have a thorough discussion about your entire physical and emotional state. You might be asked, "Is your back also hurting? Have you been under emotional stress? Are you sleeping well at night? What are you eating? How is your digestion?" Then, the treatment would address you as a whole person. This philosophy takes into account the concept of synergy: that is, that the whole is somehow greater than the sum of its parts. This, in turn, implies that you cannot treat one part of a person without affecting the other parts. In other words, we are unlike automobiles. On a car, if the tires go bald, it's obvious that you need to change the tires. With the human body, if your arm hurts, it may be because your back is out of alignment and pinching on a nerve that ultimately reaches your arm; thus, it wouldn't work to replace your arm. And taking a painkiller would only alleviate the symptom, but not the cause.

The second major philosophy is Mechanism, also known as Rationalism. Modern medicine, or allopathic medicine, is based on the philosophy of Mechanism: dissect the whole into its parts and understand the chemistry of the parts, in order to treat those individual parts. The

Mechanistic approach involves scientific research, drug research and testing, and the lab work (blood tests, urinalysis, scans, etc.) that physicians use to monitor a patient's health. So, when you have a fever, an allopathic physician might take your temperature, check your pulse, your blood pressure, perhaps even do a blood test, and based on the final diagnosis, he or she may recommend that you take acetaminophen, or antibiotics, or just get a good night's sleep.

The medical historian, Harris Coulter, maintains that the pendulum of power has swung between these two philosophies of medicine for over 2,500 years, with Mechanism dominating for the better part of the last century. There has always been this struggle between holistic practitioners and allopathic practitioners, as though the two concepts were somehow inherently incompatible. I maintain that this isn't true. At the crux of the apparent conflict between Vitalism and Mechanism is the fact that:

- Mechanists choose to focus on the small questions because the whole picture seems too great to understand all at once; whereas,
- Vitalists, faced with the same challenge, choose to make generalities about the whole picture.

Surely by now we should realize that it's simply not appropriate or productive for these two camps to fight with each another. There is so much to be gained by these two camps' coming together. A fresh perspective is what's needed.

It's altogether possible that Vitalism can benefit by taking a closer look at the big picture; and equally possible that Mechanism has been focusing on the wrong questions in the first place. In the previous chapter, we discussed the difference between studying aging (biogerontology) and studying the disease process (geriatric medicine). In light of that conversation, having the wrong focus might explain the current state of healthcare. If we had chosen to look at the roots rather than the fruits, then perhaps we would never have created the drug industry, as we know it today. In fact, later in the book, we'll see how it's possible for a Mechanistic approach to have a Vitalistic twist: studying aging at the cellular level, from the perspective of prevention, has provided answers about slowing down the aging process in the entire body.

With prevention as the focus, again we're forced to ask, "Are we overusing pharmaceuticals?" Pharmaceutical theory is very much justified in trying to understand a particular reaction in the body, and then creating a chemical that can manipulate that reaction in a desirable manner. Meanwhile, additional effects (side effects) on the body are duly ignored, as long as the drug can create a therapeutic result for some acceptable amount of time. Simply put, if we feel sick and we can take a medicine that makes us feel better without dropping dead that day from the side effects, we will continue to take that drug. Yet, there is not a drug manufactured that does not have a list of side effects, as necessarily disclosed by the manufacturing companies themselves; and at least some of these side effects will eventually catch up with us with continued use. In addition, besides what is disclosed by the pharmaceutical companies at the time of product release, there are an alarming number of drugs that have had additional severe side effects that have caused them to be pulled off the shelf.

As a mother, it is terrifying to think about the possible consequences of giving medications to my toddler; not only for fear of unknown side effects, but because I can never know what any of these chemicals is really doing in the long run. For instance, there are numerous over-the-counter cold/allergy and fever medications, including some for children, which have had to be recalled because they contain Phenylpropanolamine (PPA). PPA is also present in some dietary and weight control supplements. Disturbingly, it has been found to increase the risk of hemorrhagic stroke in women, according to an article in the New England Journal of Medicine (Kernan et al., 2000). FDA officials estimated PPA might cause between 200 and 500 hemorrhagic strokes per year in patients, ages 18 to 49. You may recognize, and hopefully no longer find on the shelf, the following brand name medications that at least at one time contained Phenylpropanolamine:

Acutrim Diet Gum Appetite Suppressant Plus
   Dietary Supplements
Acutrim Maximum Strength Appetite Control
Alka-Seltzer Plus Children's Cold Medicine Effervescent
Alka-Seltzer Plus Cold medicine (cherry or orange)
Alka-Seltzer Plus Cold Medicine Original
Alka-Seltzer Plus Cold & Cough Medicine Effervescent
Alka-Seltzer Plus Cold & Flu Medicine Effervescent
Alka-Seltzer Plus Cold & Sinus Effervescent
Alka-Seltzer Plus Night-Time Cold Medicine Effervescent
BC Allergy Sinus Cold Powder
BC Sinus Cold Powder

Comtrex Deep Chest Cold & Congestion Relief
Comtrex Flu Therapy & Fever Relief Day & Night
Contac 12-Hour Cold Capsules
Contac 12 Hour Caplets
Coricidin D Cold, Flu & Sinus
Dexatrim Caffeine Free
Dexatrim Extended Duration
Dexatrim Gelcaps
Dexatrim Vitamin C/Caffeine Free
Dimetapp Cold & Allergy Chewable Tablets
Dimetapp Cold & Cough Liqui-Gels
Dimetapp DM Cold & Cough Elixir
Dimetapp Elixir
Dimetapp 4 Hour Liquid Gels
Dimetapp 4 Hour Tablets
Dimetapp 12 Hour Extentabs Tablets
Naldecon DX Pediatric Drops
Permathene Mega-16
Robitussin CF
Tavist-D 12 Hour Relief of Sinus & Nasal Congestion
Triaminic DM Cough Relief
Triaminic Expectorant Chest & Head Congestion
Triaminic Syrup Cold & Allergy
Triaminic Triaminicol Cold & Cough

Besides such extreme cases, when we start to suffer a side effect from the medication we're taking, we might choose to take yet another pill down the road to combat that side effect, if one is available; and so the vicious cycle continues. It reminds me of the time my husband got into a major crash on his roller blades and ended up in the hospital emergency room. The doctor gave him some very strong pain medication, which upset his stomach. Within minutes, he was offered something for his stomach. The whole staff was dumbfounded when my husband refused the stomach medication, as well as additional painkillers. He had decided that he would rather bear the pain than fill up on pills. His unexpected refusal may have been due, in part, to a study I had recently shared with him on what happens to people when they end up in the hospital. In April of 1999, the *Journal of the American Medical Association* published a study on adverse drug reactions in hospitals. The authors concluded that by one interpretation of the statistics, adverse reactions to medications taken within the confines of a hospital as directed by physicians were the 4th leading cause of death in the country. Even by a more conservative interpretation of the statistics, adverse drug reactions within hospitals would still be the 6th leading cause of death (Lazarou et al., 1998). Also important to note is that the researchers only included the cases where drugs were properly prescribed, and ignored any instances of misuse. That is, these numbers do not represent a lack in the quality of care these patients received. Rather, these findings are

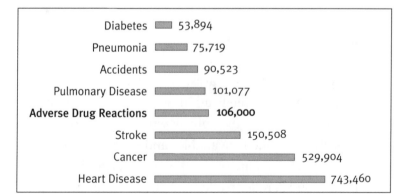

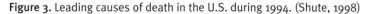

Figure 3. Leading causes of death in the U.S. during 1994. (Shute, 1998)

disturbing because they *do* represent how the cure can often be worse than the illness.

Adverse drug reactions generally come in two varieties:

- The first stems from "too much of a good thing," as in the case of blood pressure becoming too low through excessive medication.
- The second consists of unknown side effects, such as liver damage caused by the common painkiller acetaminophen.

People can usually take over-the-counter and prescription pills without experiencing acute problems; but extrapolating from the extreme situation of dying from adverse drug reactions, we must realize that our health will be challenged every time we introduce these strong chemicals into our bodies. *It should give us great pause to think that after stroke, heart disease and cancer, the next big killer is adverse reactions to drugs as administered in hospitals.* If nothing else, it should raise questions about the general acceptance of using pharmaceuticals as the norm for treating disease. Looking at the chart on page 42, we might well reconsider the level of attention we give to eliminating adverse drug reactions (106,000 deaths per year) versus improving highway safety (90,523 deaths per year due to accidents). Yet FDA funding for policing drugs once they are in the marketplace is a mere $9 million, as compared to the $160 million annually authorized by the U.S. Government for highway safety grant programs (Report number 0003-9926, 2001).

You may have been surprised to learn that adverse drug

reactions in hospitals are responsible for more deaths than highway accidents. A report published by The Institute of Medicine, an independent research group, would suggest that the adverse drug reaction statistic represents only one category on a list of fatal medical errors that are occurring in our hospitals on a regular basis (Ricks, 2001). Further investigation is obviously warranted; there is not enough research currently being conducted that deals with this disturbing subject.

Even sparser are studies in relation to children, which too often lag behind adult studies. As a mother, I'm influenced by general recommendations aimed at parents by various regulatory agencies. For instance, on long road trips, I'm sometimes tempted to take my screaming child out of the safe hold of her car seat in order to console her; but I dare not. I wonder, then, how I would react if a regulatory agency of some sort were to advise me never to take my child to a hospital. I say this because a recent study revealed that the most typical medical mistake made with infants and small children is what's known as a "tenfold error," where a decimal point gets misplaced on the written order for a medication. A recent, fatal, tenfold error was that of a child getting 5.0 milligrams of a painkiller instead of the intended 0.5 milligrams. How often does this happen? Dr. Rainu Kaushal, an internist and pediatrician practicing in Boston, worked with a research team in order to find an answer. Their data showed that within a six-week period, 616 mistakes were made out of a total of 10,778 written orders for medication at Children's Hospital Boston and Massachusetts General Hospital. Twenty-six of these mistakes were serious and eighteen were potentially fatal

(Kaushal et al., 2001). Granted, I may end up having to take one of my children to a hospital at some point. But, I also wonder how many hospital visits could be avoided just by extending the practice of preventative medicine to include our children as well. This alone could go a long way toward reducing the incidence of tenfold error.

Another disturbing trend is the increase in pharmaceutical advertisements—in print, on radio and television, and on the Internet—introducing new diseases, in need of new drugs. These ads are slick, but I still have to wonder, "Which came first, the drug or the disease?" Just the other day I saw an advertisement for a drug that introduced Premenstrual Dysphoric Disorder, or PMDD, which is apparently distinct from Premenstrual Syndrome, or PMS. PMDD symptoms include irritability, sadness, sudden mood changes, tension and bloating. I've decided that it's an even split for me. Six months of the year, I have PMS; the other six, I have PMDD.

On a more serious note, I am not alone in wondering, "Which comes first these days, the drug or the disease?" The public is becoming cynical about new diseases that were not heard of a generation ago; thus, when researchers are trying to study complicated diseases like Attention-Deficit Hyperactivity Disorder, or ADHD, they must do so in a climate further complicated by controversy. The topic of debate can be summed up by this pointed question: "Did the diagnosis of ADHD become defined by the invention of a new drug?"

I recently saw a report on public television on this very

subject and found myself wondering what is really known about ADHD. Is ADHD a "new" disorder? According to Professor Russell Barkley, who has been studying ADHD since the 1970s, the syndrome has been observed since the early 1900s. Also, research suggests that it is a highly inheritable disease, and autopsies on people with ADHD have revealed a distinct difference in a small area of their brains.[2] However, this information does not provide a sure-fire way to test for ADHD (Smith, 2001). There are so many unanswered questions; it is not surprising that the public is wary.

At the same time, there are some questions that seem obvious, but are not being asked! It's interesting to note that most of the children shown in the PBS documentary were eating junk food; and yet, how is it that there was not a single parent or expert who seemed to be concerned about this? I have to wonder if they even consider the macaroni and cheese, pizza, fruit punch, etc. that those kids were eating to be junk food? They failed to ask the most obvious, and perhaps the most important, question of all:

"What is the role of nutrition in the prevention and management of ADHD?"

Later, we'll discuss in depth how critical nutrition is for the development and maintenance of our brains. But for now, let me say that in light of new research on prenatal care, it also becomes clear that nutrition during pregnancy can play a critical role in the prevention of ADHD and other diseases. Even when there is a history of ADHD in the family and a genetic marker is found, environmental and lifestyle

---

[2] The posterior inferior vermis of the cerebellum is smaller in ADHD brains.

factors can always attenuate genetic dispositions.

Finally, some experts are concerned that the public is being misled to believe that all emotional and behavioral problems are really chemical imbalances that are treatable by medication. The pharmaceutical companies argue that drugs are highly effective in these situations. This attitude scares me. If we, as a society, are conditioned to give highly addictive drugs to our children with the attitude, "Hey, the drug works, my child behaves better, does better in school, etc.," then where do we draw the line? What is our incentive to look at other factors, such as stress and nutrition?

One worrisome development is that some misguided, albeit well-meaning, teachers are handing out literature about ADHD in the classroom for their students to take home, and are encouraging the use of highly addictive drugs, like Ritalin, for treatment. All too often, pharmaceutical companies with vested interests are providing this literature, as well as funding researchers, policy makers, and even self-help groups. Furthermore, these pharmaceutical companies heavily solicit doctors; until recent legislation, some doctors were being offered as much as $100 to talk to a pharmaceutical representative for as little as 15 minutes about Adderall, a newer drug used to treat ADHD.

Even when we're sure about the diagnosis of a disease, the drugs being used to treat them are still in question. We have to ask ourselves, "Do drugs really provide cures? Or do we simply suppress the symptoms and sometimes trade one ailment for another? For instance, take my personal case of using ibuprofen regularly for muscle pain. It wasn't too long before I got an ulcer, which is a common side effect of ibuprofen. In fact, in trying to find a particular situation where a drug has actually provided long-term relief without side effects, I have to rack my brain for a reference. The only examples that come to mind are certain metabolic diseases that are treated with various sugars and dietary supplements; but then again, these are not really drug therapies, per se.

On the other hand, I can fill a book with references to drugs that have complications, contraindications and disappointing results. Short of doing that, I'll comment on two general situations. The first is our growing reliance on over-the-counter medications and what consequences that may have. The second is our inability to successfully use drugs to combat some of the deadliest diseases that plague the people of the United States.

Let's look first at our love affair with pill popping. What happens when we get a cold or flu? How many of us sit and wait for it to pass versus making a short trip to the drug store and self-prescribing acetaminophen, ibuprofen, decongestants or, at least, some aspirin? After all, the TV ads promise a good night's rest and a smile at work the next day. The reality is that these common cold medications actually suppress the immune system at the very time when we need the immune system to be fully engaged in resisting infection. The very symptoms we are trying to alleviate are a critical part of the body's attempt to expel foreign microbes.

It's important to note that cold and fever medications

are not the promise of a quicker recovery from the infection. A double blind, placebo-controlled study was conducted on healthy individuals to test the effects of over-the-counter drugs such as aspirin, acetaminophen and ibuprofen against placebo on virus elimination, immune response and common cold symptoms (Graham et al., 1990). Sixty healthy subjects were infected with a virus and given aspirin, acetaminophen, ibuprofen or placebo (a neutral sugar pill). By carefully monitoring virus elimination, antibody levels, clinical symptoms and signs, and blood leukocytes, the researchers could determine the severity and duration of the infection. In summary, the study showed that the cold medications suppressed the subjects' immune systems, *increased* infection-time and the level of respiratory discomfort.

Since these cold medications prolong the duration of a cold or flu, then why do we persist in taking these drugs? One reason may be that we're not comfortable with letting the immune response run its course in fighting off the infection. That is, we don't appreciate the war going on inside us as our immune systems are making antibodies and eliminating cells infected by viruses, fungi, bacteria or parasites. We just want to go to work without a headache, runny nose or general malaise, even though these are simply symptoms of an immune system hard at work. Chances are that we won't die if we pop a decongestant and show up at work; yet, there are many costs to this approach. The immune system exhausts many of the body's reserves for the energy and raw materials it needs in order to fight the infection. And, if we stress the immune system longer than we need to, then we're taking energy and raw materials away from the normal maintenance and upkeep of the rest of the body's machinery. This can contribute to premature aging of the body, including an immune system that works less efficiently later on. Thus, taking drugs now for a cold will not only slow down our ability to fight that cold now, but will also affect our ability to fight the next cold. In addition, these over-the-counter drugs come with the risk of long-term side effects. Remember, for example, that acetaminophen can cause liver damage. Is the risk really worth it? My grandfather used to say that if you take something for your cold, it'll last seven days and that if you do nothing, it might take a whole week.

We may have a choice about taking medications when we catch a cold, but what about more severe health problems that require professional care? I'm reminded again of my father's heart attack. The drug Propranolol is often prescribed after myocardial infarctions to prevent further damage to the heart and to regulate the heart beat. I often encouraged my father to eliminate the need for the drugs prescribed for him by taking on healthy lifestyle habits instead. He would say, "Come on, I'm *not* overweight. I stopped smoking after the heart attack and I do exercise." While I acknowledged the changes he had made, I was convinced that they weren't sufficient to prevent a second heart attack. For one reason or another, most people don't make sufficient lifestyle changes when faced with challenges to their health; instead, they continue filling their prescriptions, as if taking a drug were the most important preventative measure. Unfortunately, my father was no different.

In a double blind study where patients were given

Propranolol or placebo, the death rates were actually reduced by 50% among patients who took Propranolol. This would seem to be an overwhelmingly positive result, except for the fact that death rates were also reduced by 50% for those taking a placebo (Shivkumar et al., 1998). To top it all off, one of the possible contraindications of the drug Propranolol is that it has been shown to induce cardiac failure. When my father eventually passed away, it was as the result of cardiac failure. While this does not mean that taking Propranolol was the cause of his heart's failing, it is ironic to me that he was taking a drug whose potential side effect is the same as the precise potential outcome we were trying to avoid.

The Propranolol study is a great example of the "placebo effect," where the very act of undergoing treatment, such as seeing a doctor or taking a pill, helps the patient to recover. The placebo effect may be the reason why doctors are still willing to prescribe antibiotics to patients who demand medicine for the viral infection we call the common cold, even though antibiotics are useless against viruses. I believe that the placebo effect is the single most important reason we are in love with popping pills.

The placebo effect works often enough to encourage us to overuse pharmaceuticals. I'm not the only one who thinks this is the case. Dr. Walter Brown of Brown University Medical School has been studying the placebo effect for two decades. In an article for *Scientific American*, he writes:

> Some studies, including one by the U.S. Office of Technology Assessment, suggest that only 20% of

modern medical remedies in common use have been scientifically proved to be effective; the rest have not been subjected to empirical trials of whether or not they work and, if so how. It is not that these treatments do not offer benefits; most of them do. But in some cases, the benefit may come from the placebo effect.... The very effectiveness of a placebo is troublesome to us doctors and to other medical experts. It impugns the value of our most cherished remedies, it hampers the development of new therapeutics and it threatens our livelihood (Brown, 1998).

While most of the scientific and medical community, as well as the general public, may view the placebo effect as trickery or false science, Brown doesn't subscribe to this derisive assessment of the placebo effect. He says that although a drug may not have pharmacological activity, it can still be powerful in treating illness. Furthermore, Brown thinks that doctors could do more to incorporate bedside manners that enhance the patient's confidence and sense of control over the situation, all of which can enhance the placebo effect. He even suggests that doctors could actually prescribe placebos as an alternative to strong medications.

Brown's example of the use of placebos in the treatment of high blood pressure was of particular interest to me. My mother has had to take expensive blood pressure medication for over a decade and the side effects have been severe, especially over time. Brown reports that in a study using antihypertensive agents vs. placebo, the success rate of using placebo alone was 25% (Materson et al., 1993). While the investigators' motives were to study the antihypertensive agents, Brown suggests that with a 25% success rate, placebos should be used first, as an alternative, in order to see if hypertension could be controlled without expensive, strong medications. Perhaps physicians will be able to successfully incorporate the positive benefits attainable from the placebo effect. Some people believe the practice of homeopathic medicine to be the ultimate utilization of the placebo effect. Approved by the FDA, but not strictly monitored, homeopathic remedies are considered drugs; and yet, they have not met the approval of the scientific community as having a real chemical effect. So, the next time you have a cold or minor illness, you might ask your homeopath to suggest a remedy for you. See if it does you some good, albeit perhaps only from the powerful placebo effect.

The placebo story has yet another twist in relation to pharmaceuticals. Some scientists believe that we are putting stronger medications on the market because of placebo-controlled studies. Stronger drugs have stronger side effects; so when patients feel these side effects, they know that they have the real drug; this in turn may trigger a placebo response making the medication more powerful than it might be otherwise. If this is in fact the case, then double blind studies are rarely blind, and we may be selecting drugs that are more toxic and less effective.

My discussion on the placebo effect wouldn't be complete without mentioning some recent evidence suggesting that we've put too much weight on the placebo effect to begin with. Two Danish scientists examined more than 100 studies involving 8,500 patients and found little evidence to support the notion of a placebo effect. They concluded that while the placebo effect can have some benefit, when it comes to serious illnesses such as cancer, heart disease or the disability of stroke, the "mind-body connection" that is currently popular in alternative medicine, is not going to be enough to overcome these serious illnesses (Bailar, 2001; Hrobjartsson and Gotzsche, 2001). While this study may be suggesting that the "mind-body connection" isn't sufficient to overcome serious illnesses, it doesn't totally overturn the long-observed phenomenon of the placebo effect. That is, this study doesn't prove that taking a placebo won't yield any results at all.

Finally, I'm left doubting all the studies ever done with pharmaceuticals, given the questions surrounding the placebo effect:

• Are treatments, in fact, more effective because of the placebo effect?
• Does the placebo effect promote the selection of stronger drugs?
• Does the placebo effect actually exist, and if so, to what extent does it work?

And, in light of these unsettling doubts, I'm still left with the bigger question: "Why do we routinely use pharmaceuticals when they carry the risk of severe side effects?" The obvious answer seems to be that many people would rather pop a pill than start exercising and eating better. If a pill can give immediate results, why work so hard? Surprisingly, it's recently been shown that even moderate lifestyle changes can be more effective than the latest designer drugs for the prevention of Type II diabetes. A

Diabetes Prevention Program was conducted over a three-year period at 27 centers with more than 3,000 participants between the ages of 25 and 85. Given that some 10 million Americans are currently at high risk for getting adult-onset (Type II) diabetes, a great many people stand to benefit from this landmark finding: *lifestyle changes can be more effective than drugs.* And the lifestyle changes don't have to be dramatic either. Walking 30 minutes a day and dropping an average of 15 pounds can cut the risk of Type II diabetes by 58%. Compare this to a new state-of-the-art diabetes pill called metformin, which reduces the risk by only 31% (Medical News, 2001). It seems that we have accepted the widespread use of pharmaceuticals as part of our Default Health Program without asking, let alone answering, this crucial question. Study after study suggests that it is past time for us to look more closely at alternatives to traditional drug therapy, and to end our love affair with pill popping. Now, I'm not suggesting that those of you who are currently on medication should suddenly stop. What I'm advocating instead, is that you:

- Carefully read the rest of this book.
- Consider your potential for becoming drug-free.
- Consult with your doctor about your decision to reduce or eliminate medications by substituting healthy lifestyle changes.
- Seek out other health professionals who can help you to create a treatment program that emphasizes nutrition, stress management and exercise.
- Continue to make the healthy choices that will hopefully allow you to avoid, reduce or eliminate any unnecessary

dependence on pharmaceuticals.

Drug-Free America—is it just a pipe dream?

*"If one is lucky, a solitary fantasy can totally
transform one million realities."*
—Maya Angelou

In the pages of this chapter and again in *Chapter Eleven,* I've shared my own views and research of the current scientific literature on pharmaceuticals. If you would like to gain another perspective, I would recommend a recent book called *Over Dose: The Case Against the Drug Companies,* by Jay S. Cohen, M.D. (Tarcher/Putnam, 2001). Dr. Cohen is an associate professor of family and preventative medicine at the University of California, San Diego. Among other things, he talks about "the poor research methods on the part of the drug companies" and "the deliberate effort to create easy, one-size-fits-all dosages that both appeal to doctors and produce inflated effectiveness statistics."

Again, I want to state that it has been my observation that most centenarians do not own a pillbox. When I looked for scientific data that might indicate a correlation between longevity and the use of pharmaceuticals, I was unable to find any research studies. I guess we'll just have to let the centenarians speak for themselves.

4

Designer Genes

An insidious aspect of the Default Health Program is our tendency to blame disease on our genes. As I've told you, my father suffered from heart problems, like his ancestors before him; so, I suppose I should just resign myself to my fate and forgo any attempt at a healthy lifestyle. When my time comes to suffer the inevitable, I'll just have to trust pharmaceuticals and the latest techniques in medical therapy. I know that they have already developed very sophisticated surgical methods that utilize remote-controlled micro-instruments; they no longer have to make huge incisions in order to clean one little clogged artery. Surely, I can count on even more advances by the time my turn comes.

While I may subconsciously think this way about the fate of my health, the fact remains that hereditary traits linked to degenerative diseases such as cancer, heart disease and stroke have only been tracked for two generations or so. Perhaps, if we could go back a hundred generations and look at these traits with a more historical perspective, we might then be able to make a more conclusive statement;

but, at present, it behooves us to look further for the causes of disease.

Each of us has a unique genetic code, which is the blueprint used by the body to express itself. These genes encode the enzymes that are made in every cell, in every tissue and in every organ. The term we use to describe the encoding of genes into enzymes is "gene-expression." The enzymes, in turn, catalyze all the chemical reactions that take place in the body. The heart's pumping, the muscles' flexing, and the brain's processing of input from our senses—these functions are all the result of enzymatic reactions. If we are suffering from a disease, then certainly some of our enzymes are not performing as they should. Since it's our genes that encode these enzymes, much of current research is focused on looking for common mutations in those who suffer from the same particular disease.

The promise of this line of research is three-fold. If we can determine which gene is failing us, we might be able to:

1) alter that mutated or dysfunctional gene in some way in order to alleviate the problem (gene therapy);
2) learn more about the disease and be able to develop better pharmaceuticals; or, at the very least,
3) let people know their risk factors for disease based upon their particular genetic codes.

This sounds great, but is it the best approach? It is possible that, in addition to "faulty" genes, other factors may actively contribute to the development of disease. For instance, there is an impressive amount of research suggesting that our environment and lifestyle play a bigger role in causing disease than our genes. So, is it fair for taxpayers to continue to fund grants for studies that concentrate on gene therapy? For instance, if our environment and lifestyle play a significant role in our health, then a doctor might treat a disease by replacing a bad gene with a good one, only to have the good gene go bad in time, as a result of the persistent, unhealthy environment and lifestyle. On the positive side, if our environment and lifestyle play significant roles in our health, must we merely suffer from certain genetic predispositions, or do we have more control than we think?

If faulty genes are the cause of modern diseases, can we track such dysfunctional genes back to prehistoric times? James V. Neel, a prominent geneticist at the University of Michigan, has said: "We could more efficiently get rid of heart disease, cancer, arthritis, diabetes, obesity and other chronic diseases by changing our diet to fit our genes than by using sophisticated gene therapy" (Carper, 1998).

According to S. B. Eaton, an anthropologist at Emory University, our genes have been around since the Stone Age. "The nutritional patterns of Paleolithic humans influenced genetic evolution during the time segment within which defining characteristics of contemporary humans were selected." That is, modern man in his industrialized environment accounts for only several hundred years, and agricultural humans for about ten thousand years, which is still a fraction of the Paleolithic human existence of 1.7 million years. He concludes, "Our genome can have changed little since the beginnings of agriculture, so, genetically, humans remain Stone Agers—adapted for a

Paleolithic dietary regimen." Our earliest ancestors were hunters and gatherers, which means that their diets were

> based chiefly on wild game, fish and uncultivated plant foods. They provided abundant protein; a fat profile much different from that of affluent Western nations; high fiber; carbohydrate from fruits and vegetables (and some honey) but not from cereals [or] refined sugars...[as well as] high levels of micronutrients and...phytochemicals (Eaton, 2000).

Once we settled into an agricultural society, we started to limit the variety of plants we ate, from hundreds down to a few dozen types. We also started to store and process our foods. With industrialization came the added complication of a fast-paced life, where convenience became a major factor in making food choices. Differences between our contemporary diets and the diets of our ancestors can have profound effects on cancer, bone mineral density and bone structural geometry, sarcopenia (the loss of lean mass with age), obesity, and insulin resistance. Eaton suggests: "Awareness of Paleolithic nutritional patterns should generate novel, testable hypotheses...and it should dispel complacency regarding currently accepted nutritional tenets" (Ibid.).

I like that suggestion. Indeed, I would advocate that we all work to "dispel complacency regarding currently accepted nutritional tenets." Such complacency is the root cause of obesity, which is one of the biggest challenges facing us today. Obesity is now an epidemic in the United States. According to a 1995 report by the Institute of Medicine,

59% of Americans meet the current definition of clinical obesity (Aldoori, 1995). With so many Americans tipping the scales, we might well ask again, "Is it our genes?" In 1962, James V. Neel proposed that in order to survive, our ancestors developed what he called "thrifty genes," that help us store fat from each feast in order to sustain us through the next famine. Hence we have the old "feast or famine" adage. So, yes, according to Neel, our genes have given us the ability to store fat; however, he says that in today's relative overabundance, the ability to store fat can become a liability.

Let's look at the case of the Pima Indians, a tribe whose progenitors split into two groups during the Middle Ages. One group settled in southern Arizona; the other moved into the Sierra Madre Mountains in Mexico. In the 1970s, the Arizona Pima Indians were forced out of farming and into the American diet. Now, they have the highest incidence of obesity reported anywhere in the world, and half of

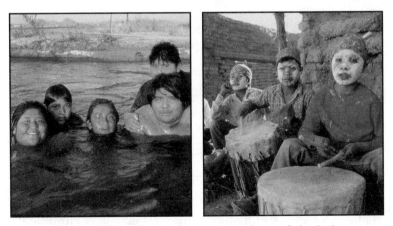

Figure 4. Effect of environment on prevalence of obesity in American and Mexican Pima Indians.
Reprinted with permission from John Annerino. Copyright ©2001.

them develop diabetes by the age of 35. It is interesting to note that the Arizona Pima Indians have an even higher rate of obesity than their white neighbors—thanks to their higher genetic susceptibility, that is, thanks to their "thrifty genes." However, the fate of the Arizona Pimas cannot be chalked up to a genetic factor alone, since their counterparts in Mexico enjoy a much different fate. As we look at these two groups of the same genetic descent today, it is difficult to recognize them as the same people. The Mexican Pimas still farm, ranch, and engage in physical labor for an average of 40 hours per week. Few have diabetes. On average, they are about 57 pounds lighter and one inch shorter than their Arizona counterparts. The fact that the Mexican Pimas remain lean shows that, even in a population with very "thrifty genes" that like to store fat, their genetic suscepti-bility does not determine their fate. Rather, environment can play the determining role (Gibbs, 1996; Ravussin, 1994). *Figure 4* on page 61 shows the impact of environment and lifestyle on genes.

Even in light of the Pima Indians study, there is still a small minority of obesity researchers who hold fast to the notion that genetic factors *alone* determine our fate when it comes to obesity. Their conclusion is based in large part on a study that included 514 pairs of twins who were separated during childhood and subsequently grew up in very different family environments. The twins were tracked over the course of their entire lives and, unlike the Pima Indian tribes, were shown to have similar body mass indexes (Fabsitz et al., 1992). Since the respective environments were not identical, this result would implicate a strong genetic factor. When faced with the findings of the Pima

Indians study, these researchers reasoned that only dramatic environmental changes, such as the difference between the plains of Arizona and the mountains of Mexico, could affect our genetic propensity.

To this I would say: yes, it is, in fact, our genes that determine how much fat we can store; and yes, our genes will be with us for life, regardless of what environment we live in. The only thing that the twin study tells me, however, is that the twins may have gone to different homes, but both families were eating the same modern diet, and not a Stone Age diet. And of course, a Stone Age diet would be the dramatic difference in environment needed to keep our "thrifty genes" in check. We can certainly wait around for either random mutations or medical advances to alter our genes to fit our modern diet, but I suggest that a more prudent approach would be to alter our diet to fit our genes. To echo Eaton, let us "dispel complacency regarding currently accepted nutritional tenets." Let's stop blaming our genes and relying on medical advances to save us. Let's make a dramatic change in the American diet and we'll dramatically lower the number of Americans struggling with obesity.

We'll talk more about obesity, both cause and prevention, in later chapters; but for now, we'll look further at genes and the exact role they play in causing diseases, such as cancer. As I stated earlier in the chapter, this determination is problematic, since we haven't been collecting data long enough to know whether genetic susceptibilities or environment and lifestyle play a bigger role. This is the old "nature vs. nurture" debate. Scientists agree that currently the most valid way to resolve this dilemma is to study the differences between identical and non-identical twins. A group of scientists did just that, working with pairs of twins from Sweden, Denmark and Finland, in an attempt to understand the contribution of hereditary factors in the causation of 28 different cancers (Lichtenstein et al., 2000). They found that if your non-identical twin sister were to have had breast cancer, then the likelihood of your getting breast cancer is only 9%; and if your twin sister were an identical twin, with genes identical to your own, the risk would only increase to 13%. For prostate cancer, the risk factors between non-identical and identical twins are 3% and 18%, respectively. After the study came out, *Newsweek* quoted Dr. Robert Hoover of the National Cancer Institute as saying, "The fatalism of the general public about the inevitability of genetic effects on cancer is unfounded" (Begley, 2000). *Newsweek* also reported how difficult it is to deflate the "my-genes-did-it" hypothesis. Many cancer researchers tend to leap to the conclusion that what this study really means is that we have not yet isolated enough genes linked to breast cancer. From the American Cancer Society to the Human Genome Project, these researchers have insisted that there is a clear link between cancer and mutated genes; therefore, more research is needed to find more cancer genes and this would clearly establish that link.

Granted, the statistics of the study were not ideal because of inherent problems in trying to distinguish nature vs. nurture. Still, the conclusion—that we have not yet found enough genes—runs counter to the evidence from hundreds of studies that have looked at how cancer risk is impacted by what we eat, drink, breathe and smoke. In summary, these studies conclude that environment and lifestyle account for at least twice the risk of cancer as that of our genes (Ibid.).

In 1996, I read an article in the *Seattle Post Intelligencer* that alerted me to the work of Dr. Donald Malins, a bio-chemist, who reasons much the same way as I do on the topic of cancer. He also directly challenges the basic premise in cancer research that says that cancer can be explained by studying genes that misfire. The article states:

> If genes are the primary driving force behind all cancer...somebody needs to explain a few anomalies. Asians have a much lower incidence of breast and prostate cancer than Americans...until they move to the United States. A generation later, these Asian Americans have the same risk. 'You can hardly attribute that to genes.... Their genes aren't being changed by flying across the Pacific' (Paulson, 1996).

Malins presents evidence that cancer is not so much a result of dysfunctional genes as it is a result of widespread genetic damage caused by free radicals. Free radicals are highly charged molecules that are by-products of normal metabolism, but unless they are neutralized by antioxidants found in our diet, they cause the havoc in the human body that scientists refer to as "oxidative stress." Malins utilizes a new method for identifying structural changes in the DNA of breast tissue to make his point. Using an instrument that bounces infrared radiation off the DNA, and then analyzing the resulting signals using sophisticated mathematics, Malins is able to monitor any structural changes caused by free radicals to the DNA. He finds significant changes within the structure of the DNA as he compares normal breast tissue to metastatic breast cancer and all of the stages in between. The process of going from normal breast tissue to full-blown metastatic breast cancer, where the cancer has progressed from the original site to other parts of the body, most likely takes decades. Dr. Malins believes that oxidative stress is what causes this predictable damage to the DNA, which, in turn, eventually leads to the formation of breast cancer (Malins et al., 1998). Dr. Malins is winning converts to his theory with the corroboration of other researchers who have independently come to the same conclusion, as we'll discuss shortly.

It would seem logical that if oxidative stress were the cause of cancer, people who eat more fruits and vegetables, and therefore have more antioxidants circulating in their bodies to combat oxidative stress, would definitely have a lower risk of cancer. This is exactly what Dr. Gladys Block, a professor at the University of California, Berkeley School of Public Health, has found to be the case. She reviewed 156 epidemiological studies from around the world that had been done on diet and major cancers (of the lung, breast, colon, cervix, ovary, bladder, uterus, mouth, esophagus, pancreas and stomach). The statistically significant and almost universal finding was that individuals who had the highest consumption of fruits and vegetables had a two- to three-fold decreased risk of developing most cancers, when compared to those who had the lowest intake of fruits and vegetables (Block et al., 1992).

Dr. Bruce Ames, Professor of the Graduate School of Biochemistry and Molecular Biology at the University of California Berkeley, is one of the leading researchers in degenerative diseases and aging in the world today. He is recognized internationally for the development of the "Ames Test." The ease and low cost of this test have made it invaluable for screening substances in our environment for possible carcinogenicity. The Ames Test has been used successfully to determine which chemicals pose a threat to our cellular DNA.

Dr. Ames reported in an interview in the *Journal of the American Medical Association* that those individuals who consume the least amounts of fruits and vegetables have twice the cancer risk as those who consume the most fruits and vegetables (Ames, 1995). According to Ames and his colleagues, "Metabolism, like other aspects of life, involves tradeoffs." Free radicals, the by-products of normal metabolism, cause extensive damage to a variety of molecules in the body, such as DNA, protein and fats. This damage is the same as radiation damage and can result, over time and without a balance of antioxidants, in degenerative diseases such as cancer, cardiovascular disease, immune-system decline, brain dysfunction, and cataracts. Fruits and vegetables are the principal sources of these important antioxidants, such as ascorbate and carotenoids. Says Ames, "Low dietary intake of fruits and vegetables doubles the risk of most types of cancer as compared to high intake and also markedly increases the risk of heart disease and cataracts. Since only 9% of Americans eat the recommended five servings of fruits and vegetables per day, the opportunity for improving health by improving diet is great" (Ames et al., 1993).

In a more recent report, Ames actually compared the

damage to DNA from micronutrient deficiencies with that from radiation. He concludes: "Common micronutrient deficiencies are likely to damage DNA by the same mechanism as radiation and many chemicals. Remedying micronutrient deficiencies should lead to a major improvement in health and an increase in longevity at low cost" (Ames, 2001).

Protecting DNA is one of the central themes of my book; I stake my reputation on the premise that our health dollars are best spent on protecting the DNA which is our birthright.

While most people have heard of the "Five A Day" program for preventing cancer, the link between micronutrient deficiencies and other major diseases, such as heart disease, is often understated. In *Chapters Seven* through *Twelve* of this book, we'll concentrate on the importance of fruits and vegetables, but I'll also show you how to select items that are high in micronutrients from the other food groups. I cannot stress enough the importance of micronutrients to your health. A group of British doctors recently published a paper indicating that micronutrient deficiencies may lead *directly* to heart failure. These doctors showed that vitamins C, E and beta-carotene help protect the arterial system, vitamins B_6, B_{12} and folic acid reduce damaging homocysteine production, whereas carnitine and CoQ10 help maintain energy output. They concluded that a deficiency of certain micronutrients may play a role in the degenerative process humans undergo during heart failure (Witte et al., 2001).

While evidence continues to grow that improving our diet might make the most difference, we are still lured by the promise of a quick fix. For instance, there was much excitement when scientists at the World Alzheimer's Congress in Washington announced the possibility of developing a vaccine to treat or prevent Alzheimer's disease, a disease that concerns a growing number of people as the Baby Boomer generation matures (Marwick, 2000; Morgan et al., 2000). The vaccine research centers on a protein by the name of beta-amyloid. Found in the brain, this protein aggregates to form "amyloid plaques." Amyloid plaques, regularly found in autopsies of Alzheimer's victims, are thought to cause dementia and memory loss. It has been shown that the incidence of amyloid plaques can be reduced in mice by vaccinating them with parts of beta-amyloid protein. While this finding is certainly exciting and seems promising, even in the best-case scenario, it will be a long time before we can expect an FDA-approved vaccination for humans. Meanwhile, we know that one way to increase our odds for preventing Alzheimer's disease is to decrease oxidative stress to the brain (Markesbery, 1999; Miranda et al., 2000; Varadarajan et al., 2000). This could clearly be accomplished by something as simple as increasing our intake of fruits and vegetables.

Even though we are intrigued by interesting concepts like a vaccine for Alzheimer's, we still need to remember the big picture. We have briefly discussed that our genes encode the enzymes which are made in the body and that those enzymes, in turn, catalyze the chemical reactions that sustain life in every cell of every tissue. When our health suffers, it is usually due to the improper functioning of one or several types of these enzymes. Pharmaceuticals can often suppress the immediate symptom of discomfort that results from such dysfunction, but currently they are unable to correct the enzyme itself. Gene therapy is the promise of being able to do just that, by manipulating the gene that has encoded that defective enzyme. Gene therapy may or may not prove to be a method of healing unto itself, since there is mounting evidence that environment and lifestyle may ultimately play a larger role in the development of disease than heredity. Again, the work of Dr. Donald Malins suggests that, over the course of a lifetime, free radicals, if left unchecked, contribute significantly to the destruction of the genes in the body. It therefore behooves us to pay closer attention to environmental factors, such as what we eat, drink, breathe and smoke.

The development of gene therapy is fraught with moral and ethical questions, which will also have to be answered before such therapy is the treatment of choice. There are also practical considerations. Even if we can get a vaccine to fix our faulty genes, we know that free radicals can still damage the new genes. And so, what is to prevent one or all of those genes from going awry again? Another complication to consider is that even if we were to cure someone of one disease using gene therapy, what's to keep that person from developing some other disease down the road? For instance, if a woman were to have her breast cancer cured with gene vaccine, but didn't alter her environment, then wouldn't she still run the risk of developing heart disease or ovarian cancer or some other disease? We could be spending most of our money, effort and time trying to lick one disease at a time, when it would be more efficient to address all of the diseases at the same time—by changing our diet to fit our genes. Ultimately, longevity seems to be a gift given by our lifestyle. Imagine going to a doctor and, instead of getting a prescription, having the doctor say, "Let's make a dramatic change in your lifestyle, and if that doesn't work, you can always take drugs." Once again, let's "dispel complacency regarding currently accepted nutritional tenets." By no means do I mean to say that diet alone will fix everything; but it's certainly one of the critical changes we must make, and *can* make—regardless of how difficult we currently think that would be. Can it possibly require more time, money and effort to start a campaign to change our diet than what is currently being invested in gene therapy and drug therapy? If we can put a human being on the moon, then we can change our diets; but first, we must be thoroughly convinced that it will make the critical difference to our health. Blaming our genes doesn't really get us anywhere; and the promise of gene therapy remains simply that—a promise for the future.

5

Your Environmental Protection Act

If genetic factors are the predominant cause of disease, we must ask ourselves how the process of natural selection managed to conserve dominant genes that cause heart disease, stroke and cancer. On the other hand, it seems that we're collecting more evidence every day that environmental factors influence the development of each and every disease, and that diet alone can increase or diminish our genetic odds.

We've known for some time now that toxins in our environment have an effect on our health. Asbestos, polluted water and smoke are all known carcinogens. That is, they have the ability to alter our genes and cause cancer. Shouldn't we consider reducing the exposure of our genes to carcinogens in the environment and in our diet? The bottom line is this: if we want to beat the genetic odds, we must provide a friendly environment for our genes, so that they can be expressed into healthy, functioning enzymes. In other words, we need to pay attention to the toxins we are exposed to on an everyday basis, and learn how we can avoid them.

In my quest for longevity, I realized very early on that I couldn't afford to ignore the toxins in my own home. My family came to the United States from India, and when I was growing up we always took off our shoes when we came in the house. Today I continue to do this out of habit, and I've learned over time to pay attention to other ways that I can clean up my act and minimize my exposure to toxins.

Why is that so important to me? Simply speaking, a toxin is a molecule that can mutate genes and/or disrupt normal cellular function. Invisible to the eye, these toxins can be inhaled from the air we breathe; they can be absorbed through the skin; they can be ingested through food and drink; and they can even be created in the body, as in the case of free radicals. In the course of the next several chapters we'll cover each of these areas of risk, but let's begin by talking about the toxins we're exposed to, even in our homes, through breathing and skin absorption.

We have all seen the movies where some big industrial plant is the bad guy, dumping toxic waste into the water, and causing horrible diseases for the neighboring town folks. You may walk out of the theater either feeling blessed that you don't live in one of those towns or wondering suddenly whether there's a chemical plant near you that is up to no good right now. Truth be known, we all need to look closer to home. Recent research shows that our exposure to toxins is far greater inside our own houses.

For many years scientists and regulatory agencies have been concerning themselves with the release of toxins into the environment; but what is even more critical to study, as scientists are assessing now, is our exposure to these substances in our daily lives (Ott and Roberts, 1998). That is to say, there is an important distinction to be made between "the sources of production" and "the sources of exposure." For example, just because a toxin, such as benzene, is being produced mostly by automobile exhaust, doesn't mean that our greatest exposure to benzene comes from cars. As discussed below, our greatest source of exposure comes from smoking and household toxins.

Benzene is just one example of the innumerable volatile organic compounds that we are exposed to daily, all of which pose a threat to our health. Benzene is harmful, especially to the tissues that form blood cells. A study published by the United States Government discusses the effects of long-term exposure to benzene:

> From overwhelming human evidence and supporting animal studies, the U.S. Department of Health and Human Services has determined that benzene is carcinogenic. Leukemia (cancer of the tissues that form the white blood cells) and subsequent death from cancer have occurred in some workers exposed to benzene for periods of less than 5 and up to 30 years. Long-term exposures to benzene may affect normal blood production, possibly resulting in severe anemia and internal bleeding. In addition, human and animal studies indicate that benzene is harmful to the immune system, increasing the chance for infections and perhaps lowering the body's defense against tumors. Exposure to benzene

has also been linked with genetic changes in humans and animals. Animal studies indicate that benzene has adverse effects on unborn animals. These effects include low birth weight, delayed bone formation, and bone marrow damage. Some of these effects occur at benzene levels as low as 10 parts of benzene per million parts of air (ppm) (Chloroform, 1989).

For the sake of our health, we need to take a closer look at some of the ways in which benzene and others pollutants are able to invade our daily lives. It will help if we recognize that the main sources of the production of benzene emissions do not correlate with the main sources of harmful exposure to benzene. Benzene is present in gasoline, some household products, and is also one of about 4,000 chemicals found in tobacco smoke.

As you can see in *Figure 5*, automobile exhaust creates about 82% of benzene emissions; industry creates 14%; individual activities, including using household products, creates another 3%; while cigarette smoking only creates about 0.1% of the total benzene in our environment. In light of this information, consider that only 18% of our *exposure*

	Sources of Production	Sources of Exposure
Automobile exhaust	82%	18%
Industry	14%	3%
Individual activity	3%	34%
Cigarette smoke (including second-hand smoke)	0.1%	45%

Figure 5. Benzene emissions. (Adapted from Wallace, 1995)

to benzene is attributable to automobile exhaust, and 3% to industry, whereas 34% is attributable to individual activities, such as using common products like glue, storing paint and gasoline in basements and garages, as well as pumping gasoline into the car; and an alarming 45% of human exposure to benzene can be attributed to cigarette smoking and second-hand smoke (Wallace, 1995).

Some people are not aware that second-hand smoke poses a very real threat to our health. It's one thing to choose to smoke; it's another to take responsibility for how that choice affects others. If you're a smoker, then you've obviously read the warning on the package. But it's important for you to know that by many measures used by researchers, second-hand smoke can be *equally* hazardous to the health of the people closest to you—literally and figuratively. For instance, the health of their endothelial cells, which are the cells that line the heart, blood vessels and lymph vessels, can be measured by the degree of constriction of the arteries. If we were to measure how much your arteries constrict after you smoke, and then measure the non-smokers, who for whatever reason have opted to remain in your smoke-filled room, *the constriction would be just as bad for the non-smokers as for you, the smoker.* Smoking does irreparable damage to the circulatory system. "So why quit? The damage is already done." Well, every cigarette does more harm—to the smoker and to the un-willing victims who are inhaling the second-hand smoke. So, at the very least, the cumulative damage comes to a halt when a smoker puts down that last cigarette (Cook et al., 1986).

It's easy to feel overwhelmed and hopeless about all the

pollution in the world these days. Often it seems totally out of our control, that we are all the victims of uncaring industrialists. But if we shift our attention away from the factory smokestacks to our own activities, there are, in fact, far more significant improvements we can make in our own immediate environments. I'm now more concerned about sitting next to a smoker at a restaurant, or using household cleaners, than with what the closest industrial plants are outgassing at any given moment. Not only do I have some control over these factors, but also, they have the most direct impact on my health and the health of my family.

Benzene is only one of the myriad volatile organic compounds that threaten our health on a daily basis. For example, did you know that whenever you take a hot shower, you are most probably exposing yourself to a toxin? Chlorine has been added to the water supply in most localities in order to disinfect the water. When this water is heated, the chlorine combines with available oxygen to form chloroform. You may find yourself in a health spa, relaxing in a chlorinated hot tub, or doing the backstroke in a heated and chlorinated pool, breathing in fumes of chloroform.

Chloroform affects the central nervous system, liver, and kidneys. It was used as a surgical anesthetic for many years before its harmful effects on the liver and kidneys were recognized. Short-term exposure to high concentrations of chloroform in the air causes tiredness, dizziness, and headache. Longer-term exposure to high levels of chloroform in the air, or in food and drinking water, can affect liver and kidney function. Toxic effects may include jaundice and burning urination. The U.S. Department of Health and Human Services has determined that chloroform may reasonably be anticipated to be a carcinogen. High doses of chloroform have also been found to cause liver and kidney cancer in experimental animals (Chloroform, 1989).

What can we do to minimize our exposure to chloroform? Obviously, skipping showers isn't an option; but improved ventilation in the bathroom and a whole house water filter or shower filter can ease our daily exposure to chloroform. Since I've been using a whole house water filter, I really notice the difference when I stay in hotels, and shower in chlorinated water. I can smell what I now know is chloroform, and notice how the un-filtered water tends to dry my skin. I'm always so glad to get home to my chlorine-free water again.

A well-ventilated room can also help to protect us from another volatile organic compound—carbon monoxide. This colorless, odorless, toxic gas is the product of the incomplete combustion of carbon. Even minimal exposure can rob the body's blood supply of oxygen, which is particularly harmful for people with heart ailments; but high exposures to carbon monoxide indoors can result in death. Although detectors are available that can alert you to dangerous levels of carbon monoxide in our environment, it would be better to monitor the sources of exposure, such as poorly operated gas stoves, space heaters and furnaces.

In addition to the risk of carbon monoxide poisoning, the air we breathe carries other invisible threats to our health. Smoking, cooking, and burning candles or firewood in our homes without proper ventilation can release fine particles into the air. Exposure to elevated levels of fine particles outdoors has been linked to premature death, but the alarming fact is that our risk of exposure *indoors* is often higher than outdoors.

Even more disturbing is a study that showed indoor air to contain at least five times more, and typically 10 times more, pesticides than outside air (Whitmore, 1994). Perhaps you've been cautious about the use of pesticides in your home; you're thinking, "I don't have to worry about this one." Well, did you know that such poisons are tracked inside on our shoes or seep in through the foundations of our homes, causing a surprisingly greater exposure to pesticides than we encounter in the food that we eat. Shoes can also track in lead from the outside. These toxins then make themselves at home in the carpet. As we walk around on that carpet, we create a small cloud of particles that increases our exposure. Most people are unaware of the ubiquitous nature of indoor pollution. According to Wayne Ott, who served on the Environmental Protection Agency for 30 years, our children are at great risk because of indoor pollution:

> Toxic house dust can be a particular menace to small children, who play on floors, crawl on carpets and regularly place their hands in their mouths. Infants are particularly susceptible: their rapidly developing organs are more prone to damage, they have a small fraction of the body weight of an adult and may ingest five times more dust—100 milligrams a day on the average (Ott and Roberts, 1998).

Now, I'm not one to worry about everyday sand and dirt, or even dead skin cells. In fact, I ascribe to the theory that exposing children to dirt and microbes is good for priming their immune systems. We'll talk later about the inadvisability of maintaining a sterile home environment, but for now let me say that there is a big difference between a microbe-free home and a toxin-free home. I do concern myself with the quality of our indoor air, especially during the winter months, and with the buildup of organic toxins.

In this regard, I'd like to mention that wall-to-wall carpeting that is made from synthetic fibers can be inherently toxic; and even the finest wool or silk carpets can trap toxins. In addition, since it's just not practical to wash our carpets as often as we wash everything else in our homes, carpeting is a place where toxins can build up most. Even though we have very little carpeting in our house, I can't help thinking about my toddler and infant roaming around in that dust cloud that Ott talked about. An alternative to carpets would be to expose hard wood floors if you have them, or resurface floors with tiles or some of the newer wood alternatives, and then decorate with smaller, washable rugs. The bottom line is that wall-to-wall carpeting is not a luxury; it's a liability.

Ott also shared another alarming fact:

Each day the average urban infant will ingest 110 nanograms of benzo(a)pyrene, the most toxic poly-cyclic aromatic hydrocarbon. Although it is hard to say definitively how much this intake might raise a child's chance of acquiring cancer at some point, the amount is sobering: it is equivalent to what the child would get from smoking three cigarettes (Ibid.).

How much of this toxin exposure can be avoided? Well, a good deal of the exposure can be blamed on our need to try to sanitize our homes. We're more obsessed with microorganisms, such as the bacteria in the sink, than we are with volatile organic compounds, such as benzene and chloroform. Given a choice, I'll take a microorganism over benzene any day. The body has the ability to fight off most bacteria if we have a healthy immune system; however, the immune system itself can falter if we are constantly exposed to chemicals like benzene and chloroform. My choice comes from the faith I have in my immune system, which is the luxury of having taken good care of my health.

Furthermore, over-sanitizing our homes can contribute to the development of a weak immune system. According to Dr. Rolf Zinkernagel, a prominent immunologist, the optimum way for a child to develop immunity is by having the protection of the mother's immunity transferred during the late stages of pregnancy and through the breast milk after birth, while still being exposed to microbes from the outside world. Yet, children are not being exposed to sufficient numbers of microbes during infancy due to the development of high standards of hygiene in developed countries (Zinkernagel, 2001). Hence, children aren't starting to make their own antibodies while still under the protection of mom's milk. After they are weaned, if they should be exposed to a contagious disease such as measles or mumps, they are at risk. Their immune systems are totally unprepared for such an encounter. It's a formidable task for the immune system to be exposed to strong microbes at ground zero, with no memory of the existence of such things. If you really want to protect young children, it is imperative that you let them be exposed to low levels of microbes. You may have heard the phrase, "Let them eat dirt." I would add to that, "Start them on dirt early on—but skip the toxins." Even for adults, a low-level exposure to microbes keeps the immune system on its toes, so to speak. The immune system is much like our muscles; if you don't use it, you'll lose it.

It's difficult to be the only family on the block with a house that doesn't "sparkle." So, unaware of the true consequences of trying to sanitize our homes, we continue to over-clean. Our shirts have to be whiter than white, and so we use bleach indiscriminately. Professional men and women dry-clean their clothes, unaware of the tetrachloroethylene that they are breathing in from those clothes. Studies suggest that women who work in dry cleaning industries, where exposures to tetrachloroethylene can be quite high, have more menstrual problems and spontaneous abortions than women who are not exposed (Doyle et al., 1997).

The bad news is that high exposure over time to volatile organic compounds can result in devastating consequences. The good news is that the use of such strong chemicals to clean our clothes and our surroundings can be easily avoided. Dry cleaning is not only toxic; it's expensive. So, I was enthusiastic when home dry-cleaning kits became available. But, when I used one, the odor that remained on the clothes was far stronger than any I had experienced with professional dry cleaning. I was suspicious, and after I read the study I just mentioned, I realized that, instead of improving the situation, I was increasing my exposure to tetra-chloroethylene with home dry-cleaning kits. Now, I hand wash most things that say, "dry-clean only." The few things that I do choose to dry-clean, I bring home and remove from the plastic bags. This allows the fumes to dissipate from the clothes before I wear them. Storing dry-cleaned clothes in plastic bags has also been shown to increase our exposure to toxins (Ott and Roberts, 1998).

One simple way to clean up the air in your home is to raise houseplants. Studies conducted by the National Aeronautics and Space Administration (NASA) discovered that plants are able to absorb most common indoor air pollutants, such as benzene and trichloroethylene. They recommend that you incorporate at least one four to five foot plant for every 100 square feet. A list of plants that help purify common household toxins can be found at www.rco.on.ca/factsheet/fs_bo9.html.

In order to raise our awareness of the toxins we create ourselves within our own homes, let's consider the following excerpts from the Recycling Council of Ontario, Canada, who also reports that households are the largest single source of hazardous waste generation in Canada (3R's in the Home, 2001). It's only when we know where toxins in our homes are coming from that we can do something about it. Every time you go out to buy one of these products, just think if there's a safer alternative. I'm giving you a huge list of safer alternatives later in this chapter.

Excerpts from the Household
Hazardous Waste Fact Sheet
November, 1996

Definition: Household hazardous waste (HHW) is the residual of products used in the home that exhibit poisonous, combustible, explosive, and/or flammable properties.

Composition: These are the categories of household hazardous wastes commonly used by municipalities to separate HHW for storage and shipment:

Acids: cleaners, descaler, disinfectant, drain opener, fertilizer, metal cement, metal cleaner, photo chemicals, polish or wax, pool chemicals, rust remover, solvents.

Antifreeze: antifreeze.

Bases: adhesives, air fresheners, ammonia, cleaners, disinfectants, drain opener, glue, metal cement, paint remover/thinner, photo chemicals, polish or wax, pool chemicals, primer, sealer, solvents, toiletries, wax stripper, wood preservative.

Batteries: alkaline battery, button battery, car/vehicle battery, lithium battery, nickel-cadmium battery.

Flammables: adhesives, air freshener, alkyd paint, artist craft paint, brake fluid, carburetor cleaner, cleaners, concrete water sealer, contact cement, paint remover/thinner, de-icer, disinfectant, driveway sealer, enamel, filler, fuel, gas line antifreeze, glue, herbicide, high heat paint, inks, lacquer, linseed oil, liquid plastic, lubricants, mineral spirits, motor oil, photo chemicals, polish or wax, pool chemicals, power steering fluid, primer sealer, resin or sealer, rust or metal paint, rust remover, shoe care products, solvents, specialty paints, spray paint, stain, stucco, tar or roofing patch, toiletries, transmission fluid, undercoating, varnish, wall paper prep, water repellent, wax stripper, wood finish, wood preservative.

Gas Cylinders: fuel, propane.

Oil: motor oil, oil filters.

Other: fire suppressants.

Oxidizer: bleach, cleaners, disinfectant, fertilizer, hardener, photo chemicals, pool chemicals, toiletries.

Paint: alkyd paint, enamel, latex paint.

Pesticides: herbicide, insecticide, mixed pesticide and fertilizer, specialty paints.

Pharmaceuticals: non-prescription drugs, prescriptions, sharps (hypodermic needles).

In 1995 Canadian manufacturers produced over:

- 20,000 tons of toilet bowl cleaners
- 19,000 tons of granular detergents
- 4,000 tons of floor polish
- 4,000 tons of acid drain cleaners
- 45,000 tons of other household cleaners

Health and Environmental Concerns

Paint Products: Methylene chloride is used extensively in paint removers, and is very dangerous if heart ailment exists. Oil-based products are combustible. Latex and water-based paints don't require solvent thinners (they may still have toxic substances, but lack volatile hydrocarbon solvents).

Solvents: Solvents are fast-drying substances that dissolve something else. Breathing of these vapors or accidental drinking can be harmful or even fatal. Long-term exposure to some solvents may cause liver and kidney problems, birth defects, central nervous system disorders, and cancer. Some solvents are flammable. Avoid products containing highly toxic ingredients such as nitrobenzene, trichloroethane, dinitrobenzene (carcinogens), and oil of cedar (central nervous system stimulant).

Caustic/Corrosive: Caustic/corrosive materials are effective cleaners, but they can cause severe eye and skin damage. Any acid or alkaline product is corrosive and is also poisonous if ingested.

Aerosol Sprays: Aerosol sprays contain a high proportion of organic solvents—mist particles enter the lungs and blood stream.

Pesticides and Herbicides: Pesticides and herbicides are poisons and may cause damage to skin, eyes or internal organs; some are flammable. They contribute to environmental contamination when used improperly or in excess. Chemical fertilizers are fast-acting, short-term boosters that may deplete soil's growing capacity with extended use. May also be corrosive, flammable or toxic.

Automotive Products: Automotive Products such as motor oil, transmission and brake fluids, and antifreeze all contain hazardous chemical compounds. Antifreeze is sweet tasting and may attract children and pets; it is a poison.

Motor Oil: Used motor oil contains cadmium, lead,

benzene and polyaromatic hydrocarbons, all of which can be harmful to human health. One part per million (ppm) of used motor oil in water causes taste and odor problems. 35 ppm will create a visible slick that can affect aquatic life. 50 ppm can interfere with the proper operation of water treatment facilities.

How would you know that you might be buying something that contains hazardous chemicals? Let's go back to the Fact Sheet.

Identifying Hazardous Products

Some products might carry the labels shown below, while other products that contain only small amounts of hazardous substances may only have "hazard statements" such as:

- Keep out of the reach of children
- Do not store near food or beverages
- Avoid contact with eyes, skin and clothes

Corrosive: Substances that eat or wear away at many materials, for example, battery acid, oven cleaners, drain cleaners.

Toxic: Materials that are poisonous to you, your children and your pets, for example, rat poison, bleach, pesticides, cleaning fluids, some medications.

Reactive/Explosive: Materials that can create an explosion or produce deadly vapors, for example, bleach and ammonia pool chemicals.

Flammable: Substances that easily ignite, for example

lighter fluid, turpentine, oils, gasoline.

I would seriously consider the risks of such products before buying them. If you still decide you must use them, it's important to dispose of them properly. For instance, many people repaint their walls or cabinets, and then just throw the leftover paint remover, primer, paint, thinner, etc. in the regular trash; while, as you may have just noticed on the Fact Sheet, these items should be treated as HHWs. Another more routine example of incorrect disposal of household hazardous waste is our habit of tossing used batteries in the regular trash. Call your local hazardous waste facility to find out how to dispose of HHWs properly.

I found the Fact Sheet to be a real eye-opener. Instead of a movie like *Erin Brockovich*, where a small law firm goes after the big bad industrial plant, with a little help from Julia Roberts' cleavage, what about a movie that shows the average person going about an average day, changing some batteries in a toy for the kids and tossing the duds in the trash, picking up the dry cleaning and hanging those chemical-laden clothes in the closet, and washing down a few over-the-counter pills at the end of the day with a Jolt Cola®. Now, that's Oscar material!

Seriously, how many of the toxins we introduce into our homes could be avoided? How conscious are we about our day-to-day living and the impact it has not only on our home environments, but on Mother Earth as well? What's more important—leaving a clean planet to our children or wearing dry-cleaned suits to work so that we look good?

While there are some important choices for us to make for the sake of our health and the health of our planet, we don't have to make a choice between health and cleanliness. In fact, they go hand in hand; but most people don't realize that there are alternatives to the harsh cleaners we've become accustomed to using. For instance, used regularly, a little vinegar water will go a long way toward keeping toilets, tubs, sinks, and floors free of toxins, as well as microorganisms. Vinegar is also economical and doesn't harm most surfaces. The following is a list of safer substitutes for some household toxins also adapted from the website for the Recycling Council of Ontario. Generally, the products can be bought at the grocery store (Ibid.).

Safer Alternatives for Household Toxins

Aerosol Sprays: Use pump sprays whenever possible to replace aerosols (e.g., hair sprays).
Use fresh flowers or sachets of dried petals with spices instead of room sprays.

Bleach: Use 1 part hydrogen peroxide bleach with 8 parts water. Soak garments in this solution and rinse.

Chemical Fertilizers: (Compost) Learn how to create your own compost at home. Call your local recycling center for more information.

Chrome Cleaner: Use flour and a dry cloth.

Copper Cleaner: Pour vinegar and salt or lemon over copper and rub.

Deodorizers/Air Fresheners: Open windows or use exhaust fans as a natural air freshener. A dish of hot vinegar can get rid of fish odors. Place a small container of apple cider vinegar on a windowsill.

Baking soda placed in the refrigerator reduces odor. Fresh cut flowers or dried flower petals and spices can add a nice scent to a room. You can also boil potpourri or cinnamon and cloves in water to produce a nice scent. Insert cloves in a ripe orange and set it out on the kitchen table or hang it from the ceiling. Burn some coffee on a piece of aluminum foil on top of burner while cooking.

Detergents: (Borax) Use 1 cup of soap flakes or powder with 2 tablespoons of washing soda.

Drain Openers: Pour boiling water down the drain. Do this every week for preventive maintenance. Pour boiling water or hot water plus 1/4 cup washing soda down drain. Mix 1 cup baking soda, 1 cup vinegar and 1/2 cup salt and pour down sink. After 20 minutes, pour down a kettle of water. Use a plumber's helper (plunger) or a plumber's snake.

Fabric Softener: Adding 3 tablespoons of baking soda to the wash cycle or 1/4 cup of vinegar to the rinse cycle will soften your laundry. To eliminate static cling, toss a small wet towel in the dryer a few minutes before the cycle ends.

Floor Cleaners: Don't believe all those snazzy ads. All you need is a little soap and water. You can buy biodegradable liquid soap in most grocery stores now. Use washing soda and water.

Furniture Polish: Use 1 teaspoon lemon oil in 1 cup mineral oil, 1 tsp vinegar in a cup of water (buff with a dry cloth), or rub crushed raw nuts on wood for an oily polish. Use soft cloth and mayonnaise. For furniture that is unlacquered and unvarnished, mix 2 tablespoons olive oil, 1 tablespoon white vinegar and 1 quart warm water in a spray bottle. The polish works best when warm; heat by letting bottle sit in a pan of hot water. Rub dry with soft cloth. For furniture that does not have a protective hard coating, mix 1 tablespoon lemon oil and 1 quart mineral oil in a spray bottle. Spray on, rub, and wipe clean.

General Cleaners: (All purpose cleaner) Use 3 tablespoons baking soda, 1 cup of ammonia and ½ cup white vinegar and 1 gallon of warm water instead of the usual cleaners. Mix 3 tablespoons washing soda in one quart of warm water. Use baking soda with a small amount of water. A slice of potato removes finger prints on painted wood.

Glass and Window Cleaners: Use cornstarch and water. Mix ½ cup vinegar and one quart warm water. Wipe with newspapers. Use lemon juice with a soft cloth.

Insect Repellents: Sprinkle cream of tartar in front of the ant's path. Ants will not cross over. Cream of tartar is a substance used in baking. Place screens on windows and doors. Brewer's yeast tablets taken daily give the skin a scent that mosquitoes seem to avoid. Place eucalyptus seeds and leaves around the area where animals sleep. To repel cockroaches, use chopped bay leaves and cucumber skins, or boric acid (place carefully since one teaspoon is hazardous to animals and children). Use soapy water on leaves (then rinse), diatomaceous soil (made from shells of sea animals, available at nurseries) or ladybugs to repel insects from plants.

Mothballs: Spread newspapers around closets, or

put clothes in cedar chests, or place cedar chips around clothes.

Oven Cleaners: Salt, baking soda, water (and elbow grease). Mix 3 tablespoons of washing soda with one quart of warm water. Place liners in oven to catch any drips during baking. Sprinkle salt on spills when they are warm and then scrub. Rub spill gently with steel wool.

Paints: Share leftover paints with friends or neighbors instead of throwing them away or taking them to a hazardous waste facility near you. Water-based paints are less toxic than metal-based. After using them, no solvent is necessary for clean up.

Rat Poison: Put a screen over drains. Use mechanical-snap mousetraps. Use vitamin D.

Rug Cleaner: Sprinkle 2 parts cornmeal and 1 part borax onto carpet. Leave for one hour and vacuum thoroughly.

Scouring Powder: Dip a damp cloth in baking soda and rub. Use steel wool.

Snail/Slug Bait: Place a shallow pan with beer in the infested area. Overturn clay pots. The snails will take shelter in them during the sunny days and they can be collected and removed. Hang straws or pieces of hose near your outdoor plants. The slugs will crawl into them at night. In the morning, tap the straw or hose into a bucket of sudsy water.

Spot Removers: For grease, rub stain with a cloth dipped in borax or apply a paste of cornstarch and water. For ink on white fabric, set the fabric with cold water and apply a paste of lemon juice and cream of tartar. Let sit for one hour, then wash as usual.

Starch: Use $1/2$ teaspoon of cornstarch and 2 cups of water. Combine in a spray bottle and shake vigorously. Adjust the proportions to get the degree of stiffness you desire.

Toilet Bowl Cleaner: Use 1 cup or more of vinegar, pour into the toilet bowl then toss in a handful of baking soda. When it is foaming, scrub the toilet and flush.

You can call your local Hazardous Waste facility or Recycling Center for any additional questions you may have.

In addition to the hoard of toxic products already lining the shelves, more and more biodegradable cleaners are showing up in the marketplace. While some are "gimmicky," others are reasonable alternatives. The next time you shop, instead of grabbing the same old cleaners off the shelf, take some time to read the labels. Are you really cleaning your house? Or are you spreading health- and life-threatening toxins? Products like Simple Green®, which is a good all-purpose cleaner, can now be found in major grocery stores.

As you truly clean up your act, you'll be cleaning up Mother Earth as well. Just think of all those contaminants that you will no longer be washing down the drain. But let's face it; society isn't going to do away with disinfecting our water supply any time soon. Thus, my advice remains to filter both the water you drink and the water you shower in, and to minimize exposure to chlorinated pools and hot tubs, especially indoors. I've heard it said, "Either *buy* a water filter, or *be* a water filter." A standard urinalysis lends credence to this claim. Results show urine to be void of most of the toxins we ingest through drinking, which means the body has served as a filter by absorbing them. Some municipalities are aware of the problem and are looking to change from chlorine to some other means of disinfecting the water, such as ozone treatment.

In Seattle, the American Lung Association has begun an innovative program that trains volunteers to visit homes and help residents minimize their exposure to harmful household chemicals. Such educational programs are strengthening a universal trend toward taking greater personal responsibility for the health of our families. Right now, you are reading this book, looking for answers; and you are not alone. Certainly pharmaceuticals and gene therapy are not going to help clean up our toxic environment. It remains a necessary step that we must take for ourselves.

Here's a final note. Even when individual toxins may show no or little detectable harm, we have limited data on what the sum of all these individual toxins over the course of a lifetime may be doing to the human body. In addition, some of the repercussions of our choices may only be experienced by future generations. My rule is to take personal responsibility for my own health and the health of my family, and to avoid every toxin I become aware of as much as possible. If we're serious about achieving quality of life as we age, then we can't afford to be lazy about our personal environment. The list of household products that we've grown accustomed to using has given unprecedented momentum to the Default Health Program, not to mention the polluting of our planet. Whether it be choosing vinegar over toilet-cleaning products or hand washing over dry cleaning, I always find it to be a cathartic act whenever I can make even small changes to eliminate toxins in my home. I know it's not realistic to think that you're going to immediately incorporate all or even most of the ideas presented here. Realistically, change has to be incremental, but any and every step you take to minimize toxins in your household is an important step in the direction of better health.

6

Is your body a hazardous waste dump?

From the last chapter, we learned to look closer to home for our greatest exposure to toxins. In this chapter, we'll look even closer—inside our own bodies. Two categories of toxins are important to consider here: the toxins we ingest, and the toxins we produce as a result of metabolism. This chapter focuses on the toxins we typically ingest as a part of the Default Health Program. Both types of toxins create an unfriendly environment for our DNA to be expressed into functional enzymes. Remember that if we don't give our DNA the healthy environment it needs in order to express working enzymes, then we're bound to experience health challenges. There are various sources of toxins in and around the foods we eat:

- the containers in which foods are prepared, packaged and served
- the chemicals that are created from food processing
- the additives, such as pesticides, preservatives, and flavor and texture enhancers

Perhaps the most insidious exposure comes from the widespread use of plastic containers. While many people have some vague notion that plastic isn't as wholesome as glass or ceramic, the convenience of plastic seems too enticing to avoid. We can store leftovers in plastic containers, throw them in the microwave at work the next day, and thus feel good about the fact that we're not going out for "fast food" at lunch. Yet a whole variety of chemicals leach out of plastics and go into those healthy leftovers, especially when they're heated. Many chemicals used to make plastics mimic hormones in our body—that is, they can bind to the same receptors that our own natural hormones would bind to. Since receptors receive hormonal signals and trigger important chemical responses, the presence of these "plastic hormones" can have serious consequences. They can:

- trigger untimely chemical reactions
- be competitive inhibitors by just sitting on the receptors, so that our natural hormones can't trigger a necessary chemical reaction
- alter the number of hormone receptors by triggering too many of them and causing the body to limit receptor production

In one study, Canadian researchers showed that chemicals can leach out of the plastics used for packaging food and go into the food itself, especially after heating. This was true even of drinks that were heated in glass containers, but covered with plastic lids (Page and Lacroix, 1995).

You might be wondering why it is that we need more studies on this topic. Perhaps you've heard one of the disturbing reports in the news of the increased incidence of young girls reaching early puberty. *Time* magazine ran a feature article on this topic (Lemonick, 2000). After having read this article, I'd been mentioning these peculiar cases in my health seminars. A friend, who had recently heard me speak, called me one afternoon and told me, "Turn on *Oprah* right away!" It was on this talk show that I heard a mother relating what has to be the most stunning case I've heard—that of a two-year-old starting her menses. None of the experts on the show could pinpoint what might be causing this serious public health anomaly.

So, I got really curious and started to investigate. A hint as to a possible cause came from a study done in Puerto Rico, which has the highest known incidence of premature breast development. Researchers, who were looking for an explanation, were aware that organic[1] toxins have been shown to disrupt normal sexual development in wildlife; and that the specific toxins responsible for this disruption have been identified as pesticides and phthalates. Most of us have seen warnings about the toxic properties of pesticides; but few of us are familiar with phthalates, a group of toxic chemicals found in plastic materials. Agriculture and industry in Puerto Rico output unusually high levels of both pesticides and phthalates into the environment; thus, researchers reasoned that they should look for the presence of these toxins and their metabolites in the serum of girls with premature breast development. While no pesticides or pesticide residues were found, significant levels of phthalates were found in 68% of the girls (Colon et al., 2000).

____Phthalates are known to have estrogenic and antiandro-

---

[1] "Organic" is used here as it relates to the particular branch of chemistry—organic chemistry—that is concerned with biological molecules made up of carbon, hydrogen, oxygen and nitrogen.

genic activity; that is, they disrupt the normal activity of the androgen and estrogen hormones in the body, both of which are responsible for regulating the normal process of puberty. While the results of the Puerto Rican study do not directly implicate phthalates as the exact cause of premature puberty, they do suggest that we should at least reconsider our use of plastics. For instance, shouldn't we warn parents of the possible danger of heating infant formula in plastic bottles? In fact, I would recommend never heating up anything in plastic containers, even if the label says: "Safe for microwave use." In my mind the chemicals inherent in plastics, like other potential toxins, are guilty until proven innocent. That is, even if phthalates are not the primary culprits causing premature puberty, they are still on the "most *un*wanted list." They mimic hormones. Until we know more, why would we want to risk our health, and the health of our children, by ingesting them?

Another toxin that we may ingest unknowingly on a daily basis is aluminum. Exposure to aluminum may come from cookware, antiperspirants, baking soda, baking powder, baked goods, drinking water with high levels of aluminum near waste sites, manufacturing plants and areas naturally high in aluminum, and antacids. Aluminum causes skeletal and neurological delays in young laboratory animals, and it has been found in high levels in Alzheimer's-diseased brains (Aluminum, 1995). Aluminum is also a contaminant of commercial intravenous-feeding solutions fed to pre-term infants; prolonged intravenous feeding with solutions containing aluminum is associated with impaired neurological development (Bishop et al., 1997).

Keeping up with the latest list of potential toxins can be overwhelming when you start to read food labels. For instance, you may pick up a can of tuna to read the label and ask, "What is 'hydrolyzed vegetable protein'?" It sounds like it should be OK, since it has the words "vegetable" and "protein" in it. But in reality, it is a way for food manufacturers to disguise a food toxin (Blaylock, 2000). Caseinate is another harmful ingredient to watch for; and be on the lookout for the word "natural," which does not necessarily mean "beneficial." It pays to ask questions—"natural flavorings" could be totally innocent or totally harmful. To minimize the risk of ingesting toxins, a general approach of avoiding junk food, which I consider to be over-processed foods and most diet foods, may be the most prudent path to take. This path ends up being the one around the periphery of the grocery store, where you'll find produce, fish, meat and poultry, and a good bottle of red wine (in certain states). My advice is to avoid most of the center isles, unless you're running low on toilet paper. That's where the garden of junk food is waiting to tempt you. Have an apple instead. If you want your DNA to be expressed into functional enzymes and to avoid oxidative stress in general, "just say no" to junk food.

We'll be talking more specifically about what constitutes true junk food in *Chapter Ten*, but for now let's look at a striking correlation that is emerging. Not only does junk food contribute to oxidative stress, but it's also no accident that the huge increase in our consumption of junk food over the past decade has coincided with a huge swing to the right on America's bathroom scale. Earlier we discussed whether obesity is the result of bad genes or the environment. In an interview for *Natural Health* magazine, Kelly D. Brownell, a professor of psychology, epidemiology and public health at Yale University, tracks the evolution of the current mind-set on the issue of obesity (Fremerman, 2000). He says that we have gone through various stages:

- blaming the individual (lack of discipline)
- blaming our genes (genetic predisposition)
- blaming our lifestyle and environment (the availability of junk food, sedentary jobs, etc.)

Brownell says that while it's hard to measure the impact of personal responsibility, current estimates now attribute 25–40% of excess weight in the general population to genetic factors. This suggests that the remaining 60–75% is due to lifestyle and environment. That leaves room for some medical intervention; however, drugs for weight loss have been expensive to begin with, and, as in the case of the recall of Phen-fen and Redux, have often proved to be more dangerous than obesity itself (Brown-Beasley, 1998). In extreme situations, stomach-reducing surgery has been shown to be effective, but the procedure is expensive, painful and requires a long recovery time. It's intended as a last resort for extremely obese individuals, and certainly not as a practical solution for most overweight people (Petit et al., 2000). In addition, according to Brownell, medical intervention itself is often not powerful enough to override all the systems that are causing the problem.

We live today in what he calls a "toxic food environment." I really like this phrase because it reminds me that the food I eat has a direct impact on the environment in which my DNA will get expressed into enzymes. Brownell has coined the phrase to describe what he suggests is another explanation for the growing problem of obesity in America. We see McDonald's®, Burger King®, and other representatives of the fast food industry in the food courts of our airports and shopping malls. There are few towns that don't have at least one drive-up window and most of them are open 24 hours a day. More alarming is the fact that there are now 5,000 schools in the country that have allowed fast food franchises and soft drink machines on school premises, while, at the same time, cutting back on physical activity in the school curriculum. Brownell asks, "If you were to develop a recipe for fattening the American child, could you do better than putting fast food franchises inside the lunch room, and having soft drink machines available, and cutting back on physical activity?"

Brownell also discusses the typical serving sizes in the American diet, which are getting wildly out of hand. When Coca-Cola® got started, they bottled it in 8-ounce bottles. Thanks to progress, we can now get a 32 ounce Big Gulp® or a 44-ounce Double Big Gulp® (that's about 15 teaspoons of sugar). Brownell says, "McDonald's has...supersizes.... [We] think, oh, for only 39 extra cents, I can get the extra-big drink and extra-big fries." I would add that kids should spend a semester in school learning the difference between a garbage can, where most of this junk food belongs and our bodies, which do not need the extra 39 cents worth of food toxins. Brownell, who is open to any working solution, proposes some thought-provoking ones of his own, some of which are already in effect in a minority of cities (Fremerman, 2000):

1. Use more resources to enable the public to increase physical activity, i.e., build more bike paths and recreational centers.
2. Ban fast food and soft drinks in our schools.
3. Regulate food advertising, especially ads aimed at children.
4. Subsidize the sale of healthy foods.
5. Tax junk food.

Today the western industrialized nations share a common problem with less developed nations—malnutrition. While growing up in Kolkata, India, I saw malnutrition all around me. Then I moved to the most affluent country in the world, only to see another face of malnutrition. I was struck by the following article:

> For the first time in human history, the number of overweight people rivals the number of underweight people, according to a forthcoming report from the Worldwatch Institute, a Washington, DC-based research organization. While the world's underfed population has declined slightly since 1980 to 1.1 billion, the number of overweight people has surged to 1.1 billion. Both the overweight and the underweight suffer from malnutrition. "The hungry and the overweight share high levels of sickness and disability, shortened life expectancies, and lower levels of productivity-each of which is a drag on a country's development," said Gary Gardner, co-author with Brian Halweil of *Underfed and Overfed: The Global Epidemic of Malnutrition.* "The century with the greatest potential to eliminate malnutrition

instead saw it boosted to record levels," said
Gardner. "Often, nations have simply traded hunger
for obesity, and diseases of poverty for diseases of
excess," said co-author Brian Halweil. "Still struggling
to eradicate infectious diseases, many developing
nations' health care systems could be crippled by
growing caseloads of heart disease, cancer, and other
chronic illnesses." (Worldwatch News Release, 2000).

The toxic food environment not only introduces food
toxins into the body, but also deprives us of essential nutrients the body needs to function properly. In the past, we
may have pictured the poster child for malnutrition to be an
alarmingly thin orphan from some Third-World nation, with
bloated stomach and ribs exposed; but a new image is
emerging around malnutrition—the alarmingly obese child
in America.

Malnutrition at various stages in life is one of the main
causes of obesity; and we'll continue to explore this relationship throughout the course of the book. Unfortunately
the damaging effects of malnutrition don't stop at obesity;
the lack of essential nutrients is also a major factor in the
development of other diseases. Malnutrition can affect the
expression of genes; cause damage to enzymes, DNA, fats
and other macromolecules in the body; and, over time, it
can alter muscle mass and body fat.

Not only does malnutrition put a damper on longevity,
but it also takes its toll on the next generation. Most of
today's disease-oriented research operates from an unspo-
ken and unproven premise: our germ cells—that is, cells that

become eggs or sperms—are immune to our lifestyle habits. Such research is fueled instead by the notion that we have a genetic predisposition to disease. I maintain that, if your mother were to say to you: "Our family history shows a likelihood of cancer," there would be no statistically significant grounding to that statement. Normally, an experiment that can't be repeated and only has a few data points would get thrown out for lack of statistical significance. Were you to say, "My father had heart disease and so did my uncle," then you would only be dealing with two data points. Furthermore, you wouldn't be able to repeat the experiment for accuracy; so you really wouldn't be able to make a statistically significant statement about your genetic odds. All in all, it's hard even for researchers to track what's really going on generation after generation, because the researchers themselves are stuck with the same human lifespan as the subjects. It seems that we'll have to settle for long-term animal studies to help settle the lifestyle vs. genes debate, at least for the present.

As a matter of fact, that's what the Pottenger Cat studies set out to do in 1932. Completed in the 1942, these studies precede the current cataloging of peer-reviewed published articles, and are seldom mentioned, except in alternative medicine circles. I finally found a documentation of these studies from the Price-Pottenger Nutrition Foundation (San Diego, CA) and I bring it up here for two reasons: first, if nothing else, the experiment is brilliant in its design; and second, perhaps it may be time to repeat such a study.

In the early 1930s, Francis M. Pottenger, Jr., M.D. was using laboratory cats for studying hormones; in order to

maximize the health of the preoperative cats he fed them a
diet of raw milk, cod liver oil and cooked meat scraps. This
diet was considered by the experts of the day to be rich in
all the important nutritive substances; but the cats weren't
doing well. Dr. Pottenger noticed that they showed signs of
deficiency and a decrease in their reproductive capacity; furthermore, many of the kittens born in the laboratory had
skeletal deformities and organ malfunctions. As more cats
came into the lab, the demand for meat scraps exceeded
supply. So, Dr. Pottenger ordered raw meat scraps from a
local meatpacking plant. Because he was a diligent
researcher, he fed the raw meat scraps to a segregated group
of cats. Within a few months, the health of the raw meat
group improved. Their kittens were also in better shape. The
contrast was so apparent that it prompted Dr. Pottenger to
undertake controlled experiments. What he saw by coinci-
dence, he wanted to repeat by design. The studies he
conducted from that point on are unique; there are no
similar experiments in the medical literature. According to
the Price-Pottenger Nutrition Foundation, Dr. Pottenger
consulted with Dr. Alvin Foord, a professor of pathology at
the University of Southern California, who also served at
the Huntington Memorial Hospital in Pasadena. The foundation claims that "the studies met the most rigorous scientific standards of the day and their protocol was observed
consistently."

Using controlled experiments, Dr. Pottenger saw some
striking results. For instance, the "Raw Meat versus Cooked
Meat Feeding Experiment" showed that the cats did much
better with raw meat. One group received a diet consisting
of 2/3 *raw* meat, and 1/3 raw milk and cod liver oil. The

second group received ⅔ *cooked* meat, and ⅓ raw milk and cod liver oil. The two groups were observed for growth, skeletal development, dentofacial structures and dental health, the calcium and phosphorus content of their femurs at death, their resistance to infections, their allergic sensitivity and the ability of the females to become pregnant, deliver and nurse viable offspring.

The raw meat group fared well on all accounts. With the cooked meat group, the X-rays of facial structures showed huge variations in facial and dental structures. Even to the untrained eye, these variations were striking when compared to the uniformity of the raw meat group. The long bones of the cats that had eaten cooked meat increased in length and decreased in diameter. Other structural deformities were seen. Heart problems; nearsightedness and farsightedness; under activity of the thyroid or inflammation of the thyroid gland; infections of the kidney, liver, testes, ovaries and bladder; arthritis and inflammation of the joints; and inflammation of the nervous system with paralysis and meningitis were all common to the cooked meat group. Furthermore, these cats could hardly reproduce and when they did, their kittens were malnourished and often died within a few days (Pottenger Jr., 1995).

There were many other experiments with different food combinations, as well as switching diets to observe regeneration. The bottom line of these experiments seems to be that the more unprocessed the diet, the healthier the cats. What does this have to do with humans? Should we be eating raw meat? Well, to me these experiments raised thought-provoking questions in their day, and continue to point the way for us in the new millennium. The results suggest the need for more of these types of experiments in modern times, with modern parameters. One such parameter could be the use of modern antibiotics, as this would protect the cats from early death due to infections of the kidneys, lungs and bones. If these infections could have been elimi- nated by Pottenger, then the ultimate fate of the degenerative cats would have been more apparent. If they had lived longer, would they have developed cancers? Would they have suffered from heart failures or strokes? We really can't come to any strong conclusions about what the Pottenger studies really mean for humans; but, at the very least, they do raise an important question: what are the effects of our diet and lifestyle, not just for ourselves, but also, for future generations?

For instance, we learned from Pottenger's cats that nutrition affected not only the health and ability of the mother cat to bear kittens, but the ability of those kittens to thrive as well. Likewise with humans, the health and immune system of a mother will affect the fate of her child:

1. A woman must become immune to life-threatening infec- tious microbes before she gets pregnant in order to pass that immunity on to the child.
2. These antibodies are passed to the child through the placenta and breast milk and this process is critical to protect the child from major infections (Zinkernagel, 2001).

Thus, the quality of the very first environment that genes are exposed to after conception—the uterus—does, in fact, alter their expression. This is encouraging information for those of us on the trail of longevity. We certainly seem to be moving in the right direction: by making positive choices for our own health, we have the ability to improve not only the quality and length of our own lives, but the health and longevity of our children and future generations as well. With health in the balance, we now have incontrovertible evidence that can tip the scales: an ounce of prevention really is worth a pound of cure.

7

Express Yourself!

I find developmental biology—the study of early development from egg to birth—to be one of the most intriguing lines of research to follow. Fetal programming is an emerging field, one that might be considered a specialized field of developmental biology, since it studies the impact that gestation—the first nine months of development inside the womb—has on the body as it matures outside the uterus.

The importance of expressing the good genes

For all of us, the uterus is our first environment, and the quality of that first environment can have life-long effects on our health. The study of fetal programming is an opportunity to marvel at the miraculous workings of the body—that of the developing fetus and that of the mother. In so doing, it doesn't take long to recognize that environmental factors play an enormous role in the healthy expression of our genes. Some of the most important genes seem to get only one chance to be "turned on," and this once-in-a-lifetime opportunity occurs in the womb.

If the mother is malnourished during pregnancy, then optimal gene expression is compromised, and the fetus is programmed for a lifetime of predisposition to diseases. Hypertension, obesity, diabetes, cholesterol regulation, cancer, and allergies are just some of the disorders that may be linked to the environment in the womb. Now, here's an important disclaimer for those of us who have a tendency to put blame on others, and ourselves:

This information is not intended to serve as an example of just one more way in which your mom has failed you, nor is it to be used by moms as evidence that you haven't been the perfect mother. Nor should we use this information to judge parents who may be struggling with ill children. We're all in the learning process.

My purpose in introducing the topic of fetal programming is two-fold:

- to show how important the cell environment is for optimum gene expression
- to encourage mothers-to-be to make choices that will promote a healthy birth

Let's look at the ways in which fetal programming is a major factor behind some of our most common health problems.

Stress, High Blood Pressure, Cholesterol and Heart Disease

Ever have a very bad day, when you feel like the stress in your life is more than you can handle? We all get stressed from time to time, and when we do, it means that a class of hormones called glucocorticoids is hard at work. These hormones are responsible for the general disposition we refer to as stress. Later we'll discuss how a prolonged stressful lifestyle can seriously influence the likelihood of many disease states. But for the purpose of this discussion, let's think about how detrimental it can be for a fetus to experience the stress hormones produced when the mother is having a bad day.

One of the most miraculous examples of genetic design and ingenuity is the body's ability to block the action of stress hormones produced by the mother from reaching the fetal brain. This is done by the action of an enzyme called 11 beta-hydroxysteroid dehydrogenase (11 beta HSD); this enzyme destroys maternal glucocorticoids in the placenta before they reach the fetus. So even if Mom does get stressed out, her baby inside her remains blissfully unaware. However, if Mom is stressed, and also happens to be malnourished, then 11 beta HSD will not be expressed and the fetus will not be protected. It's a matter of economics. When the mother and fetus are living in the lap of nutrient luxury, all enzyme-making shops are open for business, resulting in an optimally healthy child. If there are few nutrients to live on, then there is only emergency power and the body is in maintenance mode, just trying to keep a viable pregnancy going. Furthermore, the baby is being prepared to adapt to an environment of famine.

In a test involving pregnant rats, even a mild restriction of protein reduced the activity of 11 beta HSD by 33% and significantly increased systolic blood pressure in the resulting offspring in early adulthood (Langley-Evans et al., 1996). This adaptation might be advantageous for the human fetus if there really were a famine and life was unduly stressful. But when the world into which a baby is born is less challenging, this fetal-programming only leaves the newborn with a lifetime disposition to cardiovascular disease (Seckl, 1998).

There may be some merit to the old wives tale: "If you think happy thoughts during pregnancy, then you'll have a happier baby, who adjusts more easily to life's challenges." When we experience something stressful, a part of the brain called the hypothalamus instructs the pituitary gland to further instruct the adrenal glands to release glucocorticoids. Then, there are feedback mechanisms that allow the hypothalamus to detect when glucocorticoid levels become too high, so that it can make any necessary adjustments. The development of this hypothalamo-pituitary-adrenal (HPA) feedback loop occurs in the fetal environment. Malnutrition, in animal studies, has been shown to lower the expression of brain corticosteroid receptors that are responsible for detecting glucocorticoid levels. The decrease in the expression of these receptors reduces the central glucocorticoid feedback regulation (Lingas et al., 1999). Less feedback regulation may explain the increase in susceptibility to stress later in life. Simply speaking, Mother Nature has given us the genes to create a mechanism for letting us know when we are getting too stressed out. But that mechanism is developed in the womb, and only if the mother is eating an adequate amount of the nutritious foods required by the fetus.

The fetal-programming of this stress-detection mechanism, the HPA, is an example of how the mother's lack of nutrition can suppress the expression of favorable genes. As we noted earlier, the stress hormones, if unregulated, can also raise blood pressure; and high blood pressure is another common disposition of adults with a history of low-birth weight (Leon et al., 1996). Now if you suspect that you're one of those individuals without the best possible HPA mechanism, don't stress out! There are many ways to compensate and you'll learn more about them as you read.

In addition to susceptibility to stress and hypertension, low birth weight also increases the risk of poor cholesterol regulation, heart disease and diabetes. Americans have been told for years to restrict their intake of cholesterol in an attempt to reduce blood cholesterol levels. That advice, as you'll learn in *Chapter Eleven*, is not well grounded in science. People should actually eat dietary cholesterol in order to better regulate blood cholesterol. Another contributing factor for poor cholesterol regulation may be fetal programming. Again, malnutrition switches the fetus to emergency mode, shunting what few nutrients are available to the most vital organ, the brain. As a result, the growth of other organs is stunted, including the liver, which is largely responsible for regulating cholesterol levels (Barker, 1997). While we have the DNA blueprint for a healthy, functioning liver, as well as for other organs, malnutrition can inhibit the full expression of those genes. Growth-stunted organs, such as a smaller kidney, can also be responsible for poor blood pressure regulation and hypertension. It's no wonder that "the link between low birth weight and cardiovascular disease is now one of the strongest in the whole field of fetal programming" (Begley, 1999).

Since heart disease is the number one cause of death in America, it makes sense that we should look more closely at the state of prenatal nutrition. To gain more insight, scientists have studied famine survivors in such faraway places as India and such distant times as the forced starvation of the Dutch by the Nazis during World War II. Still it may surprise us to find that even in America today, women are not adequately nourished during pregnancy. For instance, even mild protein deprivation can reduce the production of certain key enzymes that inhibit stress hormones from reaching the fetal brain. Protein requirements during pregnancy can average 50–70 grams a day. An example of how to meet this requirement might look like this:

Total Daily Protein Requirements for Expectant Mothers		
Meal	Typical Serving	Approx. grams of protein
Breakfast	3 eggs	20
Lunch	3 oz. fish	15
Snack	1/2 cup cottage cheese	15
Dinner	2 oz. skinless chicken	15
Total for the day		65

How many expectant mothers are getting enough protein?

Most pregnant women are used to hearing the all too common phrase: "You're eating for two now." That should be revised to: "You're eating essential nutrients for a growing fetus now." Eating for two usually translates as permission to eat excessively, such as 2 servings of pasta plus dessert, whereas what's required is quality, not quantity. While it's important to gain weight during pregnancy, women often gain too much weight, and at the same time the quality of the nutrition they receive is still lacking. Empty calories may satisfy a mother's momentary craving, but they can't replace the protein and other essential nutrients that will ensure the healthy expression of genes for a lifetime.

Diabetes

Malnutrition may also activate the genes for a thrifty metabolism. For instance, in a famine, it would be useful to have some resistance to insulin, which regulates the storage of sugar and fat in the body. After a malnourished gestation period, a baby may emerge with a resistance to insulin, as if expecting famine. Instead he or she finds the world filled with hamburgers and soda. A predisposition to diabetes is the likely result of this fetal programming of the genes (Lithell et al., 1996).

Obesity

A tragic, though brief, decline in food intake during World War II in Holland provided a unique natural experiment to study other effects of malnutrition in life after the womb. The Nazis tried to starve the Dutch population between September of 1944 and May 1945. Studies of men who were in the womb for their first trimester during this time, but got adequate food and water later in the pregnancy, show that they were born heavier, longer and with larger heads than babies who experienced normal gestation, or even babies who were in the final trimester during this forced famine. As adults, the "first trimester starved" fetuses were more likely to be obese. What may happen is this: if a fetus experiences a scarcity of food during the first trimester, the "thrifty genes" become activated. Thus, like the Pima Indians we discussed earlier, these "first trimester starved" victims must be vigilant about what they eat as adults in order to prevent obesity.

Brain disorders

The tragedy of the wartime Dutch famine has also given us valuable information about the effects of malnutrition on brain disorders such as schizophrenia and antisocial personality disorders. Severe food deprivation during the first trimester showed a substantial increase in hospitalized schizophrenia later in life for women, but not for men (Susser and Lin, 1992). On the other hand, men exposed to severe maternal nutritional deficiency during the first and/or second trimesters of pregnancy exhibited increased risk for antisocial personality disorder (Neugebauer et al., 1999). These findings suggest that early prenatal nutrition can have gender-specific effects on the risk of schizophrenia and antisocial personality disorders.

In looking for an explanation for what causes brain disorders, scientists have noted an interesting connection between brain development and body asymmetries. Fetal stress can also lead to asymmetries in feet, fingers, ears and elbows; IQs were lower in asymmetric people by as much as their physical measurements deviated from the perfect symmetry (Furlow et al., 1997). Randy Thornhill from the University of New Mexico comments that "the same stress may cause imperfections in the developing nervous system, leading to less efficient neurons for sensing, remembering and thinking" (Begley, 1999).

From these studies it's clear that during fetal development, when gene expression is the most critical, a toxic food environment can compromise normal healthy body function for life. Of course, it's still important for us to pay attention to nutrition all of our lives. Our fate is not determined either by our genes or even by our lives in the womb—they merely set the stage. William Shakespeare wrote in *As You Like It*: "All the world's a stage, and all the men and women merely players." It may seem presumptuous for me to try to expand on Shakespeare, but I'd like to suggest that, if we are to thrive, we must each take on the role of director as well.

As You Like It
Act 2, Scene 7

Jacques
    All the world's a stage,
    And all the men and women merely players:
    They have their exits and their entrances;
    And one man in his time plays many parts,
    His acts being seven ages. At first the infant,
    Mewling and puking in the nurse's arms.
    And then the whining school-boy, with his satchel
    And shining morning face, creeping like snail
    Unwillingly to school. And then the lover,
    Sighing like furnace, with a woeful ballad
    Made to his mistress' eyebrow. Then a soldier,
    Full of strange oaths and bearded like the pard,
    Jealous in honour, sudden and quick in quarrel,
    Seeking the bubble reputation
    Even in the cannon's mouth. And then the justice,
    In fair round belly with good capon lined,

With eyes severe and beard of formal cut,
Full of wise saws and modern instances;
And so he plays his part. The sixth age shifts
Into the lean and slipper'd pantaloon,
With spectacles on nose and pouch on side,
His youthful hose, well saved, a world too wide
For his shrunk shank; and his big manly voice,
Turning again toward childish treble, pipes
And whistles in his sound. Last scene of all,
That ends this strange eventful history,
Is second childishness and mere oblivion,
Sans teeth, sans eyes, sans taste, sans everything.

When we're merely actors in the play, we've let someone else usurp our power to make choices. When we reclaim the role of director, the power shifts—back to us. Perhaps in Shakespeare's time, just surviving to a ripe old age was accomplishment enough; but quantity of life means nothing without quality of life. Shakespeare's history of life ends tragically, with symptoms that sound very much like Alzheimer's disease, macular degeneration, rheumatoid arthritis or osteoporosis. Surely we can expect something better. Surely we've learned *something* since Shakespeare's time.

We have. Through all the stages of life, from beginning to end, nutrition is a key factor. We've already discussed the importance of good nutrition for the expectant mother and the developing fetus. After delivery, parents are faced with what continues to be one of the most important decisions that has to be made during the critical first year of any baby's life: breast milk or formula? Breast milk is still far from being fully understood. It's not yet possible to reproduce the dynamic and complex nature of breast milk—the composition of breast milk changes during the day, as well as with the age of the baby. The fat content in breast milk not only provides the main source of energy for the infant, but also supplies important fat-soluble vitamins, and contains essential fatty acids such as linoleic and linolenic acids. These are indispensable components of cellular membranes and are incorporated in large amounts during early brain development. We'll learn more about these essential fats later in *Chapter Eleven*. Visual acuity and development of cognitive functions are associated with the availability of these nutrients during the first year of life (Koletzko and Rodriguez-Palmero, 1999). Without breast milk, the child faces a compromised cellular environment for the full expression of desirable genes.

Some of us have no choice but to use formula for our children. When this is the case, it's especially important to supplement the formula with the essential fats that are currently lacking in most formulas made in the U.S. Actually, my recommendation would be to use goat milk, which is, by its composition, the closest substitute for breast milk (Haenlein and Ace, 1984). Depending on the child's size and tolerance, the goat milk might need to be diluted with water. In some places, you can buy goat milk from local farms. Otherwise, Meyenberg is at least one brand that is available in grocery stores nationwide.[1] Some people are also lucky enough to live in areas that have banks for breast milk, which is a wonderful resource for those who cannot breastfeed.

---

[1] You may be able to find the location of a grocery store near you that carries Meyenberg goat milk by checking their website at http://www.meyenberg.com. Again, I'd look for local farms first, as the milk may be even fresher.

Beyond the first year, the occurrence of disease in children, as well as in adults, can also be correlated to a toxic food environment. When we look at the nutritional status of children admitted into the hospital, we find that there's a high correlation between malnutrition and congenital heart disease (heart disease present at birth) (Cameron et al., 1995). A study in West Africa showed that malnourished children are also more susceptible to several infectious diseases (Man et al., 1998). Yet another study indicated that severe malnutrition is not just a problem among children, but that it's common in elderly medical admissions, and that additional nutritional depletion may occur during a hospital stay (Potter et al., 1995).

It's an American myth that malnutrition is not a problem in this country as it is in other parts of the world. It may seem as if I'm saying the obvious; of course, improved nutrition means better health. Yet most medical treatments are still based on "sick care," instead of on simple intervention methods, such as providing adequate nutrition. All too often, physicians do not even assess the nutritional status of a patient. For instance, too many children are being misdiagnosed with ADHD and being prescribed drugs like Ritalin and Adderall without a comprehensive nutritional evaluation. These drugs are among the most addictive and abused drugs that are still legal and considered as "Schedule II controlled substances" by the Drug Enforcement Administration (Novak, 2001). Yet, a simple deficit in B vitamins can have similar symptoms to those of ADHD, and can be readily treated without the risks of pharmaceuticals. B-vitamin deficiency can cause depression and anxiety in adults as well. Here again, the first step should be to check a person's diet, not to prescribe a pill.

Nutrition can also make a difference with cholesterol regulation. Poor cholesterol regulation can most certainly be dramatically improved, if not cured, through improved diet, exercise and stress reduction. Yet, too many people choose the pill option first, without ever attempting to regulate their cholesterol levels by changing their lifestyle habits. Perhaps such modification was never presented as an option; or perhaps they were not properly informed about the many side effects associated with cholesterol-lowering drugs, including death. Then again, they may have been swayed by the media hype that continues to promote these drugs. Despite all the risks, people are opting for the latest cholesterol-lowering drugs. We'll talk more about cholesterol regulation in *Chapter Eleven*.

Think about the money that we spend on sick care in hospitals. Beyond the cost of paying the doctors, nurses and administrative staff, what proportion of every hospital bill covers medical equipment and pharmaceuticals? Compare that to the part of the bill that covers the quality of nutrition in the hospital diet or the assessment of a patient's nutritional state? You get my point. Unfortunately, the Default Health Program also exists within hospital walls.

I'd like to share an extreme example of overlooking the role of nutrition in healthcare. I met a woman (we'll call her Jan) whose twin sister (Jill) had developed breast cancer and had undergone a mastectomy. Jan decided that, in light of her sister Jill's recent diagnosis and surgery, perhaps *she* should have a breast examination herself. Jan made an appointment, expressed her concerns to her doctor, and was shocked when she was advised to get a mastectomy—as a preventative measure—before she got breast cancer like her sister! This is hardly preventative medicine and must be considered an extreme intervention, especially in light of a recent study conducted on 44,788 pairs of twins in Sweden, Denmark and Finland. Published in the *New England Journal of Medicine*, this study suggests that the genetic risk factor for breast cancer, for a woman whose twin sister has breast cancer, is still only 13% (Lichtenstein et al., 2000). And even if the "Nordic Twin Study" proved to be erroneous somehow, that would still not justify suggesting a mastectomy as a preventative measure. Not only does this sound ridiculous, but also there are no studies to back up the notion that mastectomies are an appropriate treatment for the prevention of cancer.

The importance of inhibiting the bad genes

We've discussed the toxic food environment that's all around us. Eating junk food can also create a toxic food environment *within* us. Our ancient genes don't fare so well in this new toxic environment. Not only can a toxic food environment prevent necessary and desirable genes from being expressed, but it can also provide a favorable environment for unwanted genes. One devastating result of the right genes being suppressed and the wrong ones being expressed is cancer. How do cancers get started? Remember our discussion earlier about genes? The chromosomes of our cells are comprised of long strands of DNA molecules. Specific stretches of each DNA molecule—that is the genes —encode a specific sequence of amino acids. When these amino acids are thus linked together, they make the enzymes that carry out the work of the respective genes. When a gene is switched on, it gets read and the corresponding enzyme gets made in the cell. This is what occurs during gene expression. Mutations in a gene can alter the proper function of a cell by altering the amounts or the activity of certain enzymes.

For instance, the growth of cancer cells is a result of mutations to the following types of genes:

- proto-oncogenes
- tumor suppressor genes
- DNA replication and repair genes

Tumors have been found to possess mutations in one, two or all three of these classes of genes. The first two types of genes—proto-oncogenes and tumor suppressor genes—are the targets of most cancer research, since they play the important role of choreographing the life cycle of the cell. Proto-oncogenes encourage the growth and division of a cell, whereas tumor suppressor genes inhibit these processes. When mutations in proto-oncogenes cause the cell to proliferate excessively, these genes become carcinogenic (cancer-inducing) oncogenes. By contrast, when tumor suppressor genes mutate and lose their ability to suppress growth, they can contribute to cancers as well.

Tumor cells become immortal because the mutated genes ignore the normal, life cycle rules that govern the longevity of the cell. However, for cancer cells to spread, or to become malignant, cells must do more than over-stimulate their growth-promoting machinery. They must override mechanisms that normally keep them from moving into the territory of neighboring tissue. Cells usually have the ability to recognize and stay within the boundaries of the tissue in which they belong. For instance, cells in your heart tissue do not normally migrate to your lungs. Tumor suppressor genes should regulate these border patrol mechanisms.

The presence of one or even several mutations doesn't necessarily lead to cancer: even if a person has one oncogene, it does not necessarily mean that they will get cancer. Several of the border patrol mechanisms have to go awry for cancer to have the opportunity to develop, and a malignant tumor can take three or four decades of one's lifetime to develop.

In some individuals however, there's a time-compression, and they develop cancers early in life. Why is this the case? Inheritance can sometimes explain these rare early-onset cases. Typically, the mutations described above occur as a result of a lifetime of exposure to toxins introduced from the outside, as well as toxins created by the processes taking place inside our bodies. These effects occur in random cells in the body, and several random mutations have to occur to one particular cell line in order for that cell line to become cancerous. In the case of early onset, a rather rare event occurs—a critical growth-controlling gene mutation is passed on during conception. Thus, the crucial error occurred before the stem cells got a chance to fully differentiate into specific tissue type cells. As a result, the mutation got passed into many different tissues as the stem cells passed on the original mutation to *all* descendant cells.

This type of mutation results in what are called "familial cancers," and they are indeed rare. For instance, most colon cancers occur sporadically, as the result of genetic events that occur over a lifetime. One random mutation found in colon cancers silences a tumor suppressor gene called APC, and the resulting cell growth can develop into a tumor, but usually over the course of a lifetime. However, when the defective APC genes are passed from parents to children, the colonic polyps can develop rapidly, within the first 10 years of life, and in some cases become cancerous (Weinberg, 1996).

You may be thinking, "So, is it our genes after all?" First of all, most people don't inherit cancer genes; and second, lifestyle and environment are still the primary factors for most of the population. But even in the rare case of inherited cancer genes, environment will always play a role as well. Furthermore, it's a mistake to assume that all inherited mutations imply a high risk factor. For instance, when scientists discovered the oncogenes BRCA1 and BRCA2, they thought that as many as 20% of all pre-menopausal breast cancers and a substantial proportion of familial ovarian cancers could be attributed to these oncogenes. However, the Nordic Twin Study showed very low percentages for the inheritability of breast cancers (9% between non-identical twins and 13% between identical twins). Even these small percentages found between twins might be attributable to the overlooked factor of twins sharing the same environment of a mother's uterus.

Going back to fetal programming, Dr. Karin Michels and his colleagues at Harvard School of Public Health found birth weight to be a significant predictor of breast-cancer risk (Michels et al., 1996). Women who had a birth weight of approximately 5½ pounds have half the risk of breast cancers when compared to women who weighed 9 pounds, and the correlation was especially strong for breast cancers in women 50 years or younger. While this would never be a legitimate reason to starve a fetus, since that would have it's own complications, a very high birth weight may indicate a fetal environment that primes mammary tissue for cancer. Many high birth weight babies are born to obese mothers. These mothers tend to produce more growth factors such as insulin, leptin and estrogen. These excess maternal growth factors can reach the fetus and may prime fetal mammary tissue to respond to estrogen during puberty in such a way that breast cancer is promoted. Thus, the fetal environment can prime unfavorable gene expression. Certainly we need to further study what role the fetal environment might play in promoting the mutation of proto-oncogenes into carcinogenic oncogenes.

Since cancers involve mutations, it's also important to consider the importance of the integrity of our DNA repair and replication mechanisms. Genetic errors may be introduced when the enzymes that replicate DNA during cell cycling make mistakes. These are usually corrected by the DNA repair system. However, if the DNA repair system fails, then the damage becomes permanent in all descendant cells. In some rare cancers, people inherit mutations in the DNA repair system itself; but for most of the population, a functioning DNA repair system is a matter of a toxin-free environment. *A malnourished body is a toxic body.*

Among other things, a toxic body is under oxidative stress. We've talked a little about oxidative stress—where free radical toxins produced during normal metabolism can cause damage to the macromolecules in the body, including DNA. When our diets are rich in the antioxidants found in fruits and vegetables, these antioxidants can balance the production of free radicals, and all is well. However, when the free radical burden is high, then the DNA repair mechanism is outpaced by the free radical damage to the DNA.

It has been estimated that humans sustain ten thousand oxidative hits to the DNA of every cell, every day, and that damage is cumulative. This is exemplified by looking at the DNA from the lymphocytes (cells of the immune system) of the elderly, which are nine times more mutated than those of infants (Ames et al., 1993). Promising preliminary studies show that indeed the presence of antioxidants reduces DNA damage, even in the elderly. Lyophilized (dried) vegetable and fruit powders are found in a product marketed as Juice Plus+®. Juice Plus+® has been shown to increase serum levels of antioxidants (Smith et al., 1999; Wise et al., 1996). Using a laboratory analysis called a "comet assay,"

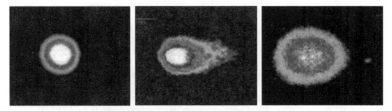

Figure 6. Typical undamaged control nuclear DNA (left); moderately damaged nuclear DNA (middle); and heavily damaged nuclear DNA (right). Images are oriented with nucleus to the right and migration of DNA to the left. Reprinted with permission from Elsevier Science; see *Selected Bibliography* (Smith et al., 1999)

researchers can determine the extent of damage to the DNA. In the comet assay, damaged DNA is broken down into small pieces, whereas undamaged DNA is relatively large. As seen in *Figure 6*, the smaller, damaged DNA spreads out easily in an electric current, giving a broad smear; the larger, undamaged pieces of DNA remain as a compact bundle.

A preliminary study showed that daily intake of these vegetable and fruit preparations reduced DNA damage by 67%; and, the data showed no apparent relationship between this finding and such factors as age, sex or smoking (Smith et al., 1999). This result holds promise for providing a friendlier environment for gene expression via a diet rich in vegetables and fruits and supplementation with vegetable and fruit concentrates.

There's another way in which fruits and vegetables

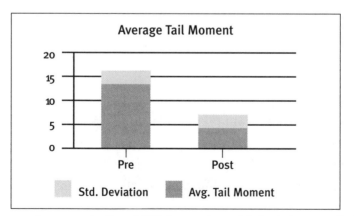

Figure 7. Average reduction of DNA damage in an elderly study group. Post-intervention with lyophilized fruit and vegetable powders show a 67% reduction as compared to pre-intervention (p<0.0001). Reprinted with permission from Elsevier Science; see *Selected Bibliography* (Smith et al., 1999)

inhibit the expression of unwanted genes. Besides being rich in antioxidants, fruits and vegetables also have other phytochemicals ("phyto" is Greek for "plant"—therefore plant chemicals) that serve as tumor suppressors. As an example, let's look at cervical cancer, which is the second most common cancer. One oncogene found in cervical cancers is called the human papillomavirus, and estrogen stimulates the growth of cells infected with this oncogene. A study using a phytochemical known as indole-3-carbinol showed that indole-3-carbinols compete for the estrogen receptor on these infected cells and reduce the expression of the culprit oncogene (Yuan et al., 1999). Another example is resveratrol, a phytonutrient found on the skin of grapes. It's considered to be one of the most effective phytochemicals for suppressing tumors, even though it is not yet clear exactly how it works (Huang et al., 1999). Indol carbinols and resveratrol are part of a growing list of powerful tumor-suppressing phytochemicals found in fruits and vegetables. Thus, while a poor diet provides a toxic environment, a diet rich in phytochemicals can inhibit the expression of unwanted genes, such as oncogenes.

Here is where we can have real control in the matter. Think of it this way. If you live long enough, your proto-oncogenes, tumor suppressor genes, DNA replication and repair genes will probably start to go south on you. And whether it's because your mom didn't eat right or whether it's because you didn't know better about household toxins until you read this book, these are now all matters of the past, which you can't change. But you could eat some broccoli and it would actually suppress the expression of these genes today. Thus, as Eaton suggested, we shouldn't be complacent about eating broccoli.

This is part of what I call the "Eating the Essentials Plan." When people try to change their diet, they all too often focus on avoiding their favorite food. Instead, if you focus on what your body absolutely needs to express the desired genes and make sure that you eat those foods first, then there will be less room in your stomach, time in your day and money in your wallet to spend on your favorite junk food.

I grew up eating lots of fruits, vegetables and legumes. Perhaps that is because kids usually like fruits, especially when there is no alternative like candy, and my mother made delicious vegetable curries and lentil dishes. The spices in curries not only enhance the flavor of food but also they serve as natural preservatives. I am thrilled that recent research shows the added advantage that many spices contain powerful phytochemicals. Some examples of tumor-suppressing phytochemicals include curcumin found in turmeric, allylic sulfides found in garlic and capsaicin in hot peppers (Chen et al., 1998; Chung, 1999; Sakamoto et al., 1997; Surh et al., 1995). For instance, curcumin inhibits various cancer processes, such as the expression of onco-genes, the growth of cancerous cells and the activity of enzymes involved in proliferation of cancer cells (Han et al., 1999; Jiang et al., 1996; Kuo et al., 1996; Lin et al., 1997). That is not to say that I think traditional curries are the best way to include more veggies in your diet. While adding the healthy phytochemicals, it's important to guard against over-cooking your vegetables, which can destroy other nutrients like fiber. However, lightly cooking your vegetables with curries could be more palatable than simply steaming them, and the spices could be more beneficial than salad dressings, which tend to be high in sugar content.

Since cancerous genes are mostly the result of a lifetime of insult to proto-oncogenes, tumor suppressor genes and the DNA repair and replication genes, it is no wonder that the American Cancer Society's top recommendations are to not smoke and to eat more fruits and vegetables. There may never be a "cure" for cancer when you consider that without eliminating the toxic environment in which cells replicate and express DNA, we will always run the risk of carcinogenic mutations. When the microscope remains focused on the promise of gene therapy or better chemotherapy or better radiation therapy, we lose sight of prevention.

With the National Cancer Act, President Nixon declared war on cancer back in 1971. Since then we have spent over 30 billion dollars on cancer research, but according to the *New England Journal of Medicine*, "the effect of new treatments and early intervention has been disappointing. The most promising approach to the control of cancer is a national commitment to prevention, with a concomitant rebalancing of the focus and funding of research" (Bailar and Gornik, 1997).

8

Radically Free

We've heard it over and over again from sources such as the American Cancer Society, the American Heart Association and the American Dietetic Association: "Evidence indicates that a diet high in fruits and vegetables may help prevent..." cancer, heart disease, premature aging—and the list goes on. But are we listening? I'd like to say the same thing one more time, but in a somewhat more radical way: *a diet lacking in phytochemicals contributes to premature death.* And this is true regardless of whether a

CATHY   By Cathy Guisewite

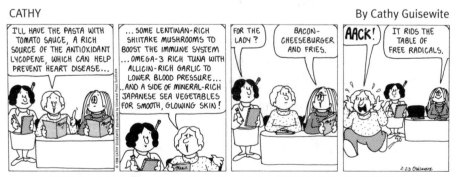

CATHY ©1998 Cathy Guisewite. Reprinted with permission of UNIVERSAL PRESS SYNDICATE.
All rights reserved.

person was conceived with perfectly fit genes, or with genetic defects, or programmed as a fetus to be more or less susceptible to disease.

The phytochemicals found in fruits and vegetables can literally mean the difference between life and death. So, when we finally decide to clean up our toxic food environment, it's not enough to get rid of the toxins in our diet; we have to be sure that it actually contains the key nutrients our bodies need in order to promote health. Some of these key nutrients cannot be manufactured in the body, but they can be supplied by the foods that we eat; we call these "essential nutrients." It was this term that inspired my "Eating the Essentials Plan" that we touched on in the last chapter.

So, let's take a look at what is really meant by the term "essential" and discuss some of the nutrients that have been officially recognized as being essential to our diet. Let's begin with amino acids; out of the twenty amino acids that serve as the building blocks for proteins in the body, nine of these are considered essential amino acids because they have to be supplied from outside the body. Two kinds of fats are also considered to be essential nutrients: linoleic acid and linolenic acid, as they are indispensable components of cellular membranes and also serve as building blocks for many important molecules like hormones. Besides these, there is a rather short list of eighteen vitamins and minerals that are also generally considered to be in the essential category. Just look on the label of One-A-Day® Essential vitamin pills if you want to get a sense of what these are:

Vitamin A	Niacin
Vitamin C	Vitamin B_6
Vitamin D	Folic Acid
Vitamin E	Vitamin B_{12}
Thiamin (B_1)	Pantothenic Acid
Riboflavin (B_2)	

This list of what are officially recognized to be essential nutrients is far too short and sadly outdated in my opinion. The bottom line is that Mother Nature's foods contain thousands of important nutrients; as science and technology progress, we learn more and more about them, give them names, try to categorize them, and study their specific roles in our health. Still we must recognize that our knowledge is incomplete about what is truly essential and what is not.

The important molecules that were discovered in the "first round" of studying food were given the name "vitamins." Along with them, we found minerals. These vitamins and minerals act as important cofactors for making enzymatic reactions work in the body. As we discovered the role of free radicals, we found that some of these vitamins also acted as antioxidants to protect the body from free radical damage. In time we began to discover that there were actually HUNDREDS of antioxidants to be found in food. Today, as science progresses further, we are finding other nutrients in food, and their roles are still being determined.

While there is much more that remains unknown than known, it's clear that we need to pay close attention to the power of Mother Nature's foods in keeping the body functioning optimally. For instance, most of the antioxidants found in fruits and vegetables still haven't been recognized officially as essential; yet the body cannot manufacture most of the antioxidants it needs in order to protect itself from oxidative stress. The various colors of produce represent different families of antioxidants: such as the orange carotenes found in carrots, the purple anthocyanins found in berries or the red lycopenes found in tomatoes. In order to thrive, we do know that the body requires the full color spectrum of antioxidants, just as it requires all of the nine essential amino acids. Yet, our Default Health Program usually consists of a diet tragically lacking in these vibrant and protective plant pigments. In this chapter, we'll discuss in more detail the importance of having the power of antioxidants on our side when it comes to confronting oxidative stress.

Whenever we burn fuel of any kind, we produce toxins.

Antioxidant Sources	Free Radical Production
• Genetic factors • Diet rich in antioxidants • Moderate exercise	• Normal metabolism • Genetic factors • Junk food • Overeating • Environmental toxins • Alcohol • Injury and trauma • Disease • Medications and treatments • Strenuous exercise • Physiological and emotional stress • Smoking • Overexposure to sunlight

Figure 8. Antioxidant Status of Humans: A Balancing Act.
If we want to guard our health, we must constantly be involved in an intricate balancing act between free radicals and antioxidants.

Think about a wood fire in your fireplace, or the gas combustion engine in your car. Burning or combustion requires oxygen; therefore this chemical process is also known as oxidation. In much the same way, our cells need to "burn" metabolites for energy. During metabolism free radicals are produced as a by-product. A free radical is a highly charged molecule that is aggressively searching for its missing electron. Free radicals can also be purposefully generated within the body for such processes as:

- *phagocytosis*: immune cells called macrophages fight infection by surrounding and consuming debris and foreign bodies with the use of free radicals
- *signal transduction*: cells perceive input and carry out necessary functions based on that input using free radicals as messenger molecules

In these processes, the production of free radicals is highly regulated and their awesome chemical power is being put to use to serve the body. What we need to focus our attention on, however, is the unregulated overproduction of free radicals. In this case, free radicals become loaded guns looking for a target, ready to harm any innocent molecule in the body that they come into contact with. You might be asking yourself, "Why would the body ever allow for the overproduction of free radicals?" That's a very good question. It may simply be because there is no free lunch. If you want to have energy then you have to play with fire. That's exactly what we are trying to do when we are producing the energy our cells need to function. Fortunately for us, we have struck a bargain on many levels with the plant kingdom. Plants are not only our breathing buddies, but they are also our eating buddies. They produce the antioxidants that can keep free radical production in check. Hence, eating like cave dwellers still remains applicable today.

Figure 8 provides a list of different ways in which harmful free radicals may be generated. These methods produce molecules such as superoxides and hydrogen peroxide. Hydrogen peroxide (H_2O_2), for example, is the product of water (H_2O) being oxidized. Can you imagine what your skin and hair would look like if suddenly the water coming out of your shower turned into hydrogen peroxide? Stripped of electrons, the molecules that make up your hair and skin would leave you dry and burned like overdone toast. The reality is that inside the body, the picture isn't much prettier, as free radicals attack our DNA, proteins and fats in order to steal electrons.[1]

So how do antioxidants protect us? An antioxidant has the power to donate an electron to a highly charged free radical—to disarm it, so to speak. How can it do this? In donating an electron, the antioxidant then itself becomes a free radical—it now has the gun. The difference is that an antioxidant radical has a much more "stable personality" than, say, hydrogen peroxide and other harmful free radicals; and in the course of a day, the body is able to flush these stable radicals out. So, when vitamin E or C donates an electron to stabilize an unstable and harmful free radical, they in turn become the stable free radicals: vitamin E radicals

---

[1]Approximately 2 to 3 percent of the oxygen used by the cells is chemically reduced by the addition of an electron and becomes a superoxide or hydrogen peroxide. Hydrogen peroxide readily permeates cellular membranes and can enter virtually all cellular compartments. In the presence of transition metals like ferrous cations (Fe^{2+}), hydrogen peroxide decomposes to become the very reactive hydroxyl free radical (.OH), which is considered to be the predominant agent of damage to macromolecules such as DNA, proteins and lipids (Weindruch and Sohal, 1997). If these macromolecules contain transition metals, then they tend to be easier targets for free radical damage.

(tocopheroxyl) and vitamin C radicals (dehydroascorbate). Another key to antioxidant protection is that they can play catch with one another, tossing an electron back and forth; thus, they can share the burden of a missing electron. "Tag! Now you're the antioxidant radical!"

We do have a limited, inborn capacity to defend against free radicals; however, it is crucial to realize that the scale is always tilted in their favor. *If we want to guard our health, we must constantly be involved in an intricate balancing act between free radicals and antioxidants.* The preponderance of free radicals leaves a trail of damaged molecules in the body. Then the body has the burden of trying to clean up the damaged molecules, by either producing new functioning molecules to replace the damaged ones, or even worse, replacing entire cells. This process exacts a huge toll from the body; we call it "oxidative stress."

Oxidative stress is now widely accepted as one of the most important contributors to aging and disease. Cells are in a continuous state of oxidative stress because of a critical imbalance: the number of free radicals being produced is greater than the body's ability to neutralize them on its own. Hence, there is a need to officially recognize antioxidants found in plant food as essential to our diet. For instance, we already discussed how free radical damage to our genes can outpace our DNA repair capabilities, unless we eat fresh, raw vegetables or fruit at every meal, preferably vegetables. While we do have some internal allies to combat oxidative stress—such as the enzyme glutathione peroxidase—for the most part, our systems are innately imbalanced without outside help.

This dependence may be one reason that some have theorized that we human beings have historically depended on eating a diet rich in the plant matter that can meet our antioxidant needs; that our very genes *require* a Stone Age diet. I certainly don't pretend to know what caused what: genes that needed antioxidants to protect them or plants that needed genes to eat them.[2] But as things stand today, it's clear that in order to live a long and healthy life, we need to eat plants.

Plants "burn" sunlight for fuel and this of course produces free radicals. Yet plants also produce a plethora of antioxidants to protect them from free radical damage. Since disease and aging are very much a matter of striking a balance between free radical production and antioxidant defenses, we should "officially" consider plant antioxidants to be essential nutrients, just as we consider certain amino acids to be essential nutrients. *Figure 8* also shows sources of antioxidants. The balance between free radical activity and antioxidant activity is often referred to as the antioxidant status in humans. More and more progressive physicians are testing their patients' antioxidant status using oxidative stress tests. I predict that in the not-too-distant future these tests will become commonplace at yearly physicals, and, perhaps eventually, as routine an indicator of health as taking your temperature or checking your blood pressure are today.

If you didn't already know before you started reading this book, you must certainly have gathered by now that free radicals damage DNA. They also wreak havoc on

---

[2] I'm thinking of a book called *The Botany of Desire: A Plant's-eye View of the World*. (New York, Random House, 2001), which promotes the idea that plants use animals to propagate the plant species.

enzymes and fats. When fat molecules, called lipids, are attacked, the oxidation process creates lipid peroxides. In common terms, we might think of these lipid peroxides as rancid fat molecules. The fat in our diet should contain important fat-soluble vitamins and essential fatty acids; the blood delivers these fat molecules throughout the body via lipoproteins. It's important to note that low-density lipoproteins (LDLs) can be modified by lipid peroxidation. While most people consider LDLs in general to be the bad guys in their cholesterol profile, it is only the *oxidized* LDLs that should be of concern. The oxidation of LDL is now accepted as a key initial event in the progression of atherosclerosis[3] (hardening of artery walls) and cardiovascular disease (Steinberg et al., 1989). Furthermore, recent studies demonstrate oxidative damage, including lipid peroxidation, to be one of the prominent features of Alzheimer's disease (Di et al., 2000; Sayre et al., 1997).

Lipid peroxidation also increases what is known as cell cycling. Cell cycling occurs when the lipids that make up the cell membrane become damaged over time. This damage prompts the chromosomal DNA of that cell to split, in order to replicate that cell, and create new cells. So what's wrong with that? Unfortunately, cells cannot replicate forever because of something called telomeres. Telomeres are found on the tips of our chromosomes and they shorten every time a cell divides. By about fifty cell divisions, telomeres disappear, and that cell then loses the ability to divide. Thus, telomeres put the ultimate limit on life expectancy. How is this process affected by oxidative stress? Oxidative stress damages membranes through lipid peroxidation and

---

[3] Atherosclerosis is a specific type of arteriosclerosis that affects large arteries, and the underlying pathologic condition in most cases of coronary heart disease, aortic aneurysm, peripheral vascular disease and stroke. Arteriosclerosis is a group of diseases characterized by the thickening of the artery wall and in the narrowing of its lumen.

increases the rate of cell cycling. In turn, there is an accompanying increase in telomere shortening and premature cell death, which results, ultimately, in a shorter lifespan.

Since our goal is to live longer and healthier lives, it's important to understand how our daily habits may contribute to cell cycling. As indicated in *Figure 8,* oxidative stress can be exasperated by:

- **Diet:** A diet lacking in vegetables and fruits is probably the most critical problem we need to address in our attempt to limit oxidative stress, since plant matter can supply most of our antioxidant needs. Eating excess calories or calories void of nutrients, such as those supplied by junk food, is yet another dietary problem worthy of our attention, since the processing of these extra or empty calories creates unnecessary free radicals.
- **Environment:** Toxins in the environment, such as nitrogen dioxide produced from automobile engine combustion, can destroy lipids and proteins.
- **Alcohol:** The consumption of most alcohols increases the oxidation of low-density lipoproteins. Excess use damages the liver and increases the likelihood of many degenerative diseases, including cancer. The exception may be moderate intake of alcohols with phytochemicals such as isoflavones and tannins as found in red wines and to a lesser extent, dark beers[4].

---

[4] In all fairness I should add that a recent finding challenges the notion that wine drinkers may get more protection than, for instance, Budweiser® drinkers. These researchers claim that socio-economic factors had been overlooked and wine drinkers tend to be in a healthier socio-economic sector to begin with (Mortensen, et al., 2001). Meanwhile, other studies suggest that one drink a day of any sort offers more health benefits than no drinks at all, because it reduces stress (Willett, 2001). And the wine-drinking scientists think that while socio-economic factors may be confounding the wine studies, red wine is still the drink of choice, because there are plenty of studies suggesting that the isoflavones and tannins found in red wine are beneficial. I like red wine; so I'm hedging my bets with one glass of red after a hard day.

- **Injury and trauma:** Tissue injury causes free radical formation by releasing heme proteins (proteins that contain iron) and transition metals, which can activate enzymes that generate free radicals. In addition, tissue injury sets off the production of mediators that lead to inflammation. During inflammation, an increase in macrophage activity is a major source of free radicals.
- **Disease and illness:** When the body is fighting a microbe or suffering from a disease, it usually means that appetite is suppressed and fewer nutrients are consumed. In addition, it's harder for the body to absorb nutrients, while the demand for nutrients is higher.
- **Medications and treatments:** Drugs can directly affect absorption, transport and utilization of nutrients, as well as suppress appetite.
- **Strenuous exercise:** Strenuous exercise is hard to define in numbers. What is strenuous for one person may not be for another. Whenever exercise exceeds a person's physical capacity, nutritional support and rest patterns, then the body will most likely produce biochemical reactions similar to acute infection and cell damage and increase the body's oxidative load.
- **Physiological and emotional stress:** Fear, grief, physiological and hormonal changes can negatively affect the antioxidant status in the body by triggering a change in appetite or by inducing chemical reactions that increase the rate of free radical production.

The above is merely a brief summary of conditions that increase oxidative stress.

The human immune system, the brain and the nervous

system are especially susceptible to oxidative stress. An immune cell, for example, has a high content of polyunsaturated fatty acids in its cell membrane, making it more susceptible to free radical damage. The cell membrane plays many critical roles for the immune system.

- It recognizes foreign molecules (antigens) that stimulate the production of antibodies.
- Receptors located in the cell membrane serve as tags for other cells of the immune system to recognize.
- Antibodies and other proteins that regulate the immune response (lymphokines) are secreted from the cell membrane.
- Once invaders have been recognized, large amounts of undamaged polyunsaturated fatty acids are needed for duplicating specialized lymphocytes trained to attack these foreign invaders (lymphocyte proliferation).
- Immune cells also have the ability to destroy other invaded cells on contact (contact cell lysis), but this capability is also dependent upon the membrane integrity.

In general, immune cells have a higher level of antioxidants as compared to other cells (Coquette et al., 1986; Papas, 1999). This higher level suggests that an immune cell needs more than its fair share of the body's available antioxidants in order for its multitude of functions to work optimally.

When we allow ourselves to passively drift into the Default Health Program we are likely to experience breakdowns in our immune systems. This is happening to so many people these days that it has become natural to expect children to get ear infections and for adults to get colds or the flu several times during the course of a year. What if, instead of taking antibiotics and cold medications that usually don't work anyway, we simply supported our immune systems by increasing our dietary intake of antioxidants? By making sure that we are vigilant about eating more antioxidant rich foods, such as vegetables and fruits, my family has, in fact, managed to stay healthy, clear out our medicine cabinet, and avoid taking antibiotics and other prescription pharmaceuticals. My little girls have never had ear infections; nor have they needed to take any of the various children's medications available on the market. Don't get me wrong. If I had a deadly bacterium or parasite roaming around in my body, I would be grateful to have an *effective* antibiotic or other pharmaceutical to combat such a bug.

However, most of the time, antibiotics and other medications are working against us in the Default Health Program. Why do I say that? Well, the lack of attention we pay to maintaining a strong immune system through diet, coupled with the overuse of antibiotics, has created a more favorable environment for microbes to thrive.

As it turns out, our most deadly foes are not lions and tigers and bears. Ever since the beginning of human existence, our most deadly foes have been microbes: viruses and bacteria and fungus. Our immune systems have been sufficient to keep the human race in existence for a long time, even though there were periods when thousands of lives were lost due to the sudden outbreak of a new kind of microbe. Yet, we've been able to survive because of the extraordinary plasticity of the human immune system—that is its ability to create antibodies for a whole universe of molecules it has never seen before. That's right! When the immune system is operating at full capacity, it can learn to fight new microbes. The immune system also has a memory, so that if a particular microbe is encountered a second time, it can respond much more quickly. Meanwhile, the microbes are constantly mutating, so that they can appear different each time they come around. When we overuse antibiotics, we force bacteria to mutate more quickly and create new strains that are resistant to the antibiotics. Couple this resistance with an immune system that is suffering from oxidative stress and slow to respond, and microbes have it made.

While antibodies are one of the greatest technical advances of mankind, their overuse is undermining their power. The Default Health Program creates a vicious downward spiral of oxidative stress, that weakens the immune system, which leads to infection, for which we take pharmaceuticals, causing further oxidative stress and more potent microbes, and so the downward spiral continues.

More long-term effects of a dysfunctional immune system include allergies, asthma, autoimmune disorders and cancer. These can be the result of oxidative stress, which mutates DNA and, therefore, challenges the function of the cells of the immune system.

In *Chapter Seven*, we discussed that lymphocytes of the elderly are likely to be nine times more mutated than those of infants (Ames et al., 1993). Two important types of immune cells, B-lymphocytes (called B-cells for short) and T-lymphocytes (T-cells) play key roles in the working of the immune system. B-cells produce antibodies to combat foreign molecules that enter the body. Antibodies constitute 20% of the proteins in the blood and the term *humoral immunity* refers to this fluid of antibodies that protect the body. You might think of your immune system as the army that protects you, and B-cells as the foot soldiers of that army. On the other hand, T-cells are more like the generals of that army. T-cells carry out *cellular immunity* by killing foreign cells and sending various instructions for other parts of the immune system to react—such as instructing B-cells to produce more antibodies. With age, cellular immunity declines as T-cells lose their full function. The generals are retiring early. As T-cells lose their function, they cannot command properly over B-cells, and as a result, humoral immunity usually rises. The foot soldiers are all geared up for war. Without proper instruction from their superiors, they get trigger-happy.

Allergies and asthma are some of the first signs of hyperactive humoral immunity—B-cells on the loose. For instance, a person suffers from allergies to pollen because his or her B-cells are over-producing antibodies to pollen, as if it were a life-threatening microbe. There are not enough T-cells around to say, "It's not the HIV virus, it's just pollen." Studies have shown that people who suffer from acute asthma attacks also have high levels of oxidative stress (Rahman et al., 1996). We also see an increase in the incidence of autoimmune disorders such as rheumatoid arthritis, scleroderma, Crohn's disease, and lupus, as people age. Individuals who have been diagnosed with an autoimmune disorder are fundamentally suffering from hyperactive immune systems that are producing antibodies to molecules of their own bodies. Oxidative stress is significantly associated with autoimmune disorders (Lisitsyna et al., 1996). You'll remember from *Figure 8* that we can support our immune systems by improving the antioxidant status of the body. We do this, in part, by eating more fruits and vegetables, by reducing stress and by following a moderate program of exercise. If we'll do our part, the antioxidants will do their job by neutralizing the potentially dangerous free radicals.

Similarly, we can delay damage to the brain by reducing the body's load of free radicals. Neurons, which are cells in the brain that process information about the world around us, have protrusions called *axons* and *dendrites* that reach out from the cell body, like long wires, in order to communicate with other cells. These axons and dendrites, like immune cells, also have fatty acid membranes vulnerable to free-radical damage. Amazingly, some axons can be as much as several meters in length. Another interesting aspect of the membranes of these wire-like protrusions, especially the dendrites, is that they are dynamic in nature—they are constantly being made and broken down, as they reach out to other cells forming short-term connections. This dynamic nature of the membrane also requires plenty of undamaged polyunsaturated fatty acids around to be used as building blocks. Vitamin E protects the lipids of membranes from oxidative damage, and vitamin E has been shown to be critical to the function of the nervous system. It is clear that one way to slow down aging in the brain is, again, to reduce oxidative stress.

Hundreds of studies also show that changing the diet to

include more antioxidant-rich foods can not only increase serum antioxidants and reduce oxidative stress, but also that such a diet can alter other physiological measures of health, such as blood pressure. In one clinical trial, 459 adults were subjected to a typical diet, low in fruits and vegetables for eight weeks, and then randomly assigned one of the following diets:

- the same diet (low in vegetables and fruits)
- a diet rich in vegetables and fruits
- a "combination" diet, rich in vegetables and fruits, as well as reduced in saturated fats

The latter two diets reduced systolic and diastolic blood pressure, with the combination diet having the greatest effect (Appel et al., 1997).

Thus, it seems that by reducing oxidative stress we should be able to reduce the dysfunctions of the immune system that lead to many of these diseases. But to date, there has been more focus on trying to lick one disease at a time. There are so many societies and associations, one for each disease, trying to raise awareness and funds for research; yet, these diseases are, at least in part, the various manifestations of oxidative stress. Studying disease from the preventative angle—of reducing oxidative stress by putting prevention into practice—has the potential benefit of protecting more people who are currently at risk from a multitude of diseases.

As mentioned, diet and moderate exercise can help us to reduce oxidative stress, but by far the greatest impact comes from diet. I related earlier that many heart patients, in trying to avoid multiple heart attacks, will continue to take pharmaceuticals, even after being made aware of their potential side effects. But these drugs do nothing to sway the balance in favor of less oxidative stress. Conversely, when researchers introduced a diet rich in antioxidants to patients who had recently had a heart attack (acute myocardial infarction), they were able to increase the patients' blood plasma levels of antioxidants, while reducing harmful lipid peroxides. Thus, diet alone can correct this delicate balance between oxidative stress and antioxidant protection, even after a person has had a heart attack. These patients were advised to eat more fruits, vegetables, soups, crushed almonds and walnuts mixed with skim milk, none of which carries the risk of side effects associated with pharmaceuticals. When compared to a control group of patients that had no change in their diet, the drop in lipid peroxides was almost five-fold for the diet-intervention group (Singh et al., 1995).

Antioxidants in fruits and veggies don't care about our genetic predispositions or our case histories; they are equal opportunity protectors of the molecules that make up the human body. Our only mission, should we choose to accept it, is to put as many of them as possible to work inside us.

Additional good news is that the power of vegetables and fruits to protect our DNA and other molecules is immediate. Yet another study tracked 28 women in order to test the hypothesis that eating more vegetables and fruits can reduce markers of oxidative cellular damage that can be assessed in blood or urine within a mere 14 days. The women increased their average daily consumption of vegetables and fruit from 5.8 servings at baseline to 12.0 servings throughout the intervention. The results of this study indicate that consumption of a diet that significantly increased vegetable and fruit intake from a diverse number of botanical families resulted in significant reductions in markers of oxidative cellular damage to DNA and lipids (Thompson et al., 1999). I should point out that I only cited a few studies here to make the point that nutrient-rich food can provide long-term protection; the importance of vegetables and fruits is not in dispute because there are plenty of studies that make this point clear. The good news is that in as little time as 7–14 days, oxidative damage to DNA and lipids can be minimized through a diet rich in antioxidants from food and by supplementation with food concentrates.

Did you have a colorful salad of broccoli, beats, carrots, tomatoes, and mixed greens as a part of your last meal? What about the meal before that? OK, how about the meal coming up? If you answered, "No" to any of those questions, you're not alone. I find it hard to do at every meal as well. But every time I eat, unless my meal includes foods rich in antioxidants, I definitely tilt the scale in favor of free radicals. Fortunately, preventative science has made another option available—we can bring things back into balance with fruit and vegetable concentrates such as those found in Juice Plus+® [5]. Pilot studies showed that regular supplementation with Juice Plus+® Orchard and Garden Blend gel caps can significantly increase serum antioxidant levels and reduce lipid peroxide levels.

After 28 days various antioxidant markers rose signifi-

---

[5] Juice Plus+® is available through local distributors, or check out their website: www.HealthWiseNW.com

cantly in the blood:

- beta-carotene by 510%
- alpha-carotene by 119%
- lutein/zeaxanthin by 44%
- lycopene by 2046%
- alpha-tocopherol (a component of vitamin E) by 58%

Meanwhile rancid fats in the blood (serum lipid peroxide levels) decreased four-fold (Wise et al., 1996), down to the detection level of the instrumentation used for measurement. Another study with elderly subjects showed that these vegetable and fruit powders improved immune regulation, concurrent with an increase in serum antioxidants (Inserra et al., 1999). I must point out here that I haven't heard of a pharmaceutical that can increase antioxidants, decrease lipid peroxidation, improve various facets of immune function, and reduce damage to DNA (as discussed in *Chapter Seven*). Furthermore, there are other studies, which I'll discuss in more detail later, showing that markers that assess the risk of heart disease also improve with vegetable and fruit concentrates. These results suggest a promising future for science and research aimed at prevention, in contrast to what has so far proved possible with disease-oriented research and pharmaceuticals.

I must point out that I'm not advocating that we continue with a diet rich in processed foods, just as long as we pop some Juice Plus+® capsules. Yes, I must admit that even that would be an improvement, as the balance would tilt further toward antioxidant protection. However, if longevity is our goal, then we need to look at the "Eating the

Essentials Plan." Yet, I will most definitely invest in supplements that make sense, are backed by research, and fill obvious voids in our diet. But these supplements mostly serve our need for micronutrients, such as vitamins and other antioxidants, minerals and other phytochemicals. There is another whole class of nutrients called macronutrients—proteins, fats and carbohydrates—that provide calories and serve as building blocks. We must make wise choices about these macronutrients as well. For instance, which is a better choice for the body's need for energy—pasta or broccoli? They're both carbohydrates; but, as you'll find out in

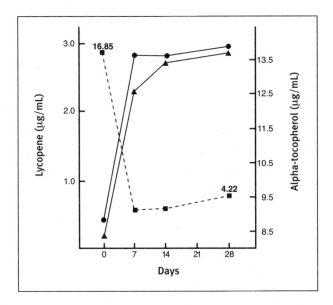

Figure 9. Plasma response of lycopene, alpha-tocopherol (vitamin E), and lipid peroxides to supplementation with dehydrated fruit and vegetable powders.

■ = lipid peroxides (nmol/mL);
● = lycopene;
▲ = vitamin E

Reprinted by permission of the publisher from Wise et al., *Current Therapeutic Research*, Vol. 57, No. 6, pp. 445-461. Copyright by Excerpta Medica Inc.

our extensive look at macronutrients in *Chapter Ten*, the right answer is definitely broccoli. The experience of real health and vitality comes when we make the choice to give the body the essentials it needs to do its job—macronutrients that are rich in micronutrients.

Meanwhile, a discussion on oxidative stress would be incomplete without touching on a topic of considerable debate: the efficacy of antioxidant supplements. The toxic food environment not only includes toxins from the foods we eat, but it also includes the toxins created inside our cells through oxidative stress. While we cannot get around the production of free radicals as we burn food for energy within our cells, we can increase our intake of antioxidant-rich foods to reduce oxidative stress. More and more experts have recognized the importance of a diet rich in antioxidants and many have written more extensive discussions on the topic than I have room for here. However, experts have yet to agree on a conclusive answer to a related question: can oxidative stress be reduced through antioxidant supplementation? Now, let me be clear that antioxidant supplementation is distinct from the supplementation with vegetable and fruit concentrates that we've discussed here. Juice Plus+® is a whole food based product and its efficacy has been proven by independent research studies and published in peer-reviewed journals. On the other hand, there are several fundamental challenges to making vitamin supplements that are as effective as food. We'll discuss these challenges and the question of antioxidant supplements when we continue our discussion in *Chapter Nine: The Great Vitamin Hoax*.

9

The Great Vitamin Hoax

Many people take vitamins. In 1998, the top thirty vitamin manufacturers alone sold a whopping $2.5 billion
worth of vitamins (Chart, 1998). That's a lot of vitamins!
But is that money well spent? For example, can vitamin
supplements reduce free radical production? The big problem here is that the whole arena of vitamins is mostly unregulated, untested and unsubstantiated, so it's difficult to
know for sure. As we've already discussed, placebo-controlled trials have proved that taking dehydrated vegetable
and fruit powders—such as those contained in Juice Plus+®—
increases antioxidants, reduces lipid peroxides, and
improves DNA repair and immune function. Other studies
indicate that isolated vitamin and mineral supplements do
not offer the same benefits as getting the antioxidants from
the complete food itself. But buyers be aware. Many isolated
supplement manufacturers are adding token amounts of
juice powders in order to make their products look appealing
to the consumer who is more interested in the label than the
content. Yet these products are not backed by research and
end up being no different from any other isolated vitamin

and mineral supplement found on the shelf.

Some healthcare providers approve testing that can identify certain nutritional deficiencies, and this can be helpful. However, this information is then used to convince people that they should use supplements, rather than as an indication of a need for a change in diet. In addition, once diagnosed, people may continue to take vitamin supplements for the rest of their lives with no follow-up test to show whether their deficiencies are being fully addressed by such supplementation.

I would agree that most people are indeed deficient in many nutrients and that we could all probably benefit from increasing our intake of nutrients; but where and how to get them is a matter of great consideration for all of us. Taking vitamin pills as cheap insurance, without knowing if they really work, may provide a false sense of security while real deficiencies continue to be ignored.

It's important for consumers, as well as healthcare providers and manufacturers, to understand that there are several fundamental challenges to the proposition of making supplements that are as effective as food. These challenges include such considerations as:

- bioavailability
- limited number of nutrients currently available in isolated form
- determining dosage
- synergistic effects between nutrients
- isomers

- multiple components of a nutrient
- localization
- determining deficiencies accurately
- claims and quality control

As a biochemist, it's impossible for me to see how any vitamin manufacturer could ever hope to overcome all of these challenges. And that is exactly what would be necessary if an isolated vitamin supplement could ever hope to be on a par with whole food.

To be perfectly frank, I never even considered the use of isolated vitamin supplements until I became pregnant. Given the technical challenges, I couldn't conceive of a vitamin pill that would be able to make up for the apples, carrots, and broccoli that might be missing in my diet. But when I became pregnant, I didn't want to presume that I had it all figured out and have my arrogance somehow get in the way of my having a healthy baby. So I started to research the efficacy of supplements, especially prenatal supplements. It seemed an ideal place to start, since one would think that prenatals should be the best supplements available. Well, remember that list of challenges? Let's see how the prenatal vitamin supplements fared, one challenge at a time, as shown by the research that I was able to find on these supplements.

Bioavailability

A supplement may say on the bottle that it has, for instance, 100 milligrams of nutrient X. However, several technical problems exist around whether the body will actually absorb and utilize that 100 mg of nutrient X. First, many binders that hold the vitamin pill together may keep the vitamin from disintegrating and from being assimilated in the gastrointestinal tract. Using the United States Pharmacopeial Convention (USPC) standard disintegration apparatus, a study of 11 products showed the disintegration time of commercially available vitamins to be highly variable (Stamatakis and Meyer-Stout, 1999).

In another study, prenatal vitamins were tested for folic acid dissolution. Among other things, folic acid has been shown to be critical for the fetal development of the neural tube, which later becomes the brain. The authors of the folic acid study concluded that only three of the nine prescription prenatal vitamins met USPC specifications for folic acid release. Not only that, most of them missed by a wide margin; for example, in two of the products tested folic acid dissolution was less than 25%. Remember those millions of dollars people are spending on vitamins? Often, they are not getting what they're paying for. These researchers also tested a wide variety of brand-name multivitamin products, all with disappointing results (Hoag et al., 1997).

Dissolution studies merely look at the ability of a vitamin to become soluble again. Beyond that, we also need to know if the vitamins can actually be found floating around in our blood serum. That is, are they bioavailable? The vitamin industry is tragically lacking in such data to back up their products. People read labels and believe that all those milligrams of this and that will actually be benefiting their bodies, when in fact, many of those milligrams won't even go back into solution, let alone be absorbed by the body.

One of the most common deficiencies to be detected is iron. That's why iron supplements are regularly recommended, especially to women of childbearing age, children and teenagers, all of whom are at risk of being low in iron. Iron supplements, however, often cause nausea, diarrhea and abdominal pain. Generally, if a person is anemic, sufficient protein is lacking in the diet, since iron is readily absorbed from meat, poultry and fish.

Even more important, though, is that bioavailability also depends on the presence of other nutrients, and supplementation of one nutrient can set off a series of other deficiencies. Of course it's important to know in prenatal care whether a women is low in iron. Often, whether there is an iron deficiency or not, women are given prenatal supplements with iron in them. This can set off a series of problems in absorbing other essential trace minerals from food sources. One study showed that prenatal iron supplements adversely influence zinc absorption during pregnancy (O'Brien et al., 2000). Whether the supplement contained iron alone or iron and zinc, the presence of iron significantly reduced the absorption of zinc (by 57%), as well as plasma zinc levels (15–25% lower) when compared to the control group. Moreover, the umbilical cord zinc concentrations were significantly related to maternal plasma zinc levels. So a mother taking an iron supplement can end up with a zinc deficiency during this critical time of fetal development.

Zinc is the second most abundant trace mineral in the body and is essential for normal growth and development in children. For example, zinc affects the taste buds, the lining of the intestines, the immune system, the retina, and it is also important to the production of sperm and testosterone. If zinc levels drop in the body, we readily absorb more zinc from meats, eggs, cheese, lentils, yeast, nuts, seeds and whole grains. However, supplementation with zinc (as well as with iron) does not make up for low zinc levels. Ironically, it interferes with the normal absorption of zinc from food, and, in addition, competes with the absorption of copper, which is essential for liver function. In another study, 40% of the prenatal supplements examined contained both iron and zinc, without a nutritionally significant amount of copper. More than 80% of the infant formulas examined had ratios of iron to copper exceeding 20:1, which is higher than the recommended ratios of 10–17:1 (Johnson et al., 1998).

Since there are many trace minerals, it is a very complicated game to try to guess how much of each trace mineral is needed in supplement form, and in what combination with other trace minerals. *Instead, the best source is adding unrefined, grey sea salt to food*[1]. Supplements can further complicate matters as iron and copper are transition metals that can increase free radical production if taken in excess through isolated supplements; however, when they are absorbed from food, iron and copper are not toxic, as they are bound to proteins in the food (Papas, 1999).

There has been much concern around calcium supplementation, mostly by women fearing osteoporosis. Calcium needs are greatest during the periods of rapid growth in childhood and adolescence, during pregnancy and lactation, and in later adult life. Ninety-nine percent of total body calcium is found in bone, and that is why calcium

---

[1]Check out www.celtic-seasalt.com as a source for unrefined sea salt.

requirements are associated with skeletal requirements. According to the National Institutes of Health Consensus Development Program (NIHCDP), "the preferred approach to attaining optimal calcium intake is through dietary sources." For most Americans, it appears that dairy products are the major source of dietary calcium because of their frequency of consumption and high calcium content (e.g., approximately 250–300 mg/8 oz milk). For those with lactose intolerance, solid dairy foods and milk with lactase enzymes may be an option. Other good food sources of calcium include some green vegetables (e.g., broccoli, kale, turnip greens, Chinese cabbage), calcium-set tofu, some legumes, canned fish, seeds, and nuts.

It seems that there are plenty of food choices for making sure we get enough calcium in our diet; yet, people still resort to antacids (e.g., Tums®) and various forms of supplements. First of all, many antacids contain aluminum, a serious toxin we discussed earlier. Overuse of antacids is clinically associated with severe renal damage and ectopic calcium deposition (milk-alkali syndrome). Other sources of calcium (e.g., bone meal and dolomite) can have significant contamination with lead and other heavy metals. It may be reassuring to someone out there that, according to the NIHCDP, "most commercial calcium preparations are tested to ensure that they do not contain significant heavy metal contamination." I personally do not know anyone who is content to voluntarily ingest any amount of heavy metal, significant or not. Other factors need to be considered around various types of calcium supplements. Iron absorption can be decreased by as much as 50% by certain forms of calcium supplements or increased by other forms that contain citrate and ascorbic acid. That sounds like a real guessing game, and neither too much iron nor too little iron absorption is desirable. Overdosing on calcium can also cause constipation and lead to kidney malfunction.

Furthermore, even the best calcium supplement requires other components in order to be effective. Without exercise, adequate vitamin D production in the body, and other dietary nutrients like magnesium (see *Figure 10*), calcium supplementation will not be enough to ward off osteoporosis. Vitamin D is also necessary in order to absorb and utilize calcium. With adequate sunlight exposure, we make vitamin D ourselves; fatty fish is another good source of vitamin D. I'll talk about the importance of exercise in the development and maintenance of bone density later, but suffice it to say that exercise is a necessary component for optimal bone structure. Also, high amounts of glucocorticoids (hormones associated with stress) decrease calcium absorption—one more reason to worry less and reduce long-term stress (NIH consensus statement, 1994).

The bioavailability problem is not limited to trace minerals. Many antioxidants are plant pigments. For instance, carotenoids are a group of over 600 different naturally occurring pigments that give plants their yellow, orange or red coloring. Of these 600, 34 have been found in human blood serum, including alpha-carotene, beta-carotene, lutein/zeaxanthin, and lycopenes. The recommended daily allowance for these relatively new antioxidants has not yet been determined. All of them seem to be important for preventing various cancers and other degenerative diseases such as macular degeneration and arthritis. It is possible to get dramatic increases in plasma levels of beta-carotene through supplementation. However, taking beta-carotene supplements reduces the body's ability to absorb lutein from food. In fact, plasma levels of lutein actually drop as a result of beta-carotene supplementation. Lycopene absorption is also subject to the presence of other carotenoids (Micozzi et al., 1992). Beta-carotene in isolation from other members of the carotenoids family may actually be harmful, as found in one study. Originally this study was designed to take place over 10 years, but was discontinued after 8 years due to an increase in the incidence of cancer and mortality rate among participants (Cancer study, 1994). Another problem is that carotenoids are fat-soluble and taking too many fat-soluble antioxidants is dangerous because, with the exception of vitamin E, they can accumulate in the liver.

Limited number of nutrients currently available in isolated form

It's important to note that the only way to get all of the 34 carotenoids that have so far been found in the blood is through diet. This is true not only for carotenoids, but also for most of the nutrients found in food. They are not found in isolated supplements. The number of nutrients found in food that are important to our health may end up in the thousands—if we ever discover them all. The number of nutrients that have already been isolated and made available in supplement form is far more limited. Most vitamin supplements contain a few dozen nutrients. Once again, only whole food or supplements made from whole food can deliver the most complete spectrum of nutrients in a balanced manner.

Dosage

The National Academy of Sciences' Food and Nutrition Board sets up the recommended daily allowances (RDAs) for essential nutrients. RDAs represent the amounts of nutrients one can expect to get by eating the recommended servings from all the five food groups of the USDA Food Guide Pyramid. (Many experts don't agree with this food pyramid, but I'll save that discussion for later.) RDAs are meant to be a measure for judging food. For instance, RDAs are used by the Food and Drug Administration to determine daily values that are required on food labels. RDAs are also used as a measure for determining standards for meals abroad for the U.S. Armed Forces. Yet, people generally relate to RDAs as if they were actually set up to be the standards by which to judge vitamin supplements. The intent of RDAs is not that they serve as a measure for vitamin supplements. The reality is that foods have nutrients for which no RDAs have been set. It is a fallacy to think that vitamins with the proper RDAs can make up for a poor diet; yet many doctors recommend vitamin supplements to people who have poor diets, while manufacturers use RDAs as a tool to justify vitamin supplements. Simply put, there is no foundation to the belief that RDAs have any correlation to vitamin supplements, particularly in light of our previous discussion on bioavailability.

Besides this incredible lack of foundation, there is constant controversy around dosage of specific nutrients, because so many factors come into play when nutrients are isolated and fragmented in the form of supplements. First, there may be contraindications (adverse side reactions) with other medications or health conditions. For instance, people with bleeding or clotting disorders should be careful about overdosing on vitamin E supplements, since it may lead to increased hemorrhaging.

It's always a guessing game when we try to reconstruct nature's food in the form of a vitamin supplement. Consider this review of prenatal vitamin and mineral supplementation:

> Available data suggest that prenatal supplements should probably contain other nutrients; pyridoxine hydrochloride, cholecalciferol, vitamin E, pantothenic acid, calcium, magnesium, zinc, copper, and possibly selenium should be considered. Interactions among the minerals and vitamins commonly found in prenatal supplements may affect the absorption of various nutrient components. Thus, very high or low levels of certain nutrients should be avoided. The chemical form of minerals should also be considered. Products should have demonstrated bioavailability for iron, zinc, and other components that are subject to bioavailability problems. Use of a low-potency product that contains a wide range of vitamins and minerals appears to be the most prudent approach to prenatal vitamin and mineral supplementation (Newman et al., 1987).

Hmm, now what is a low-potency product that contains a wide range of vitamins and minerals? Sounds a lot like a real vegetable or fruit to me. While there are a lot of "shoulds" presented in this review, I fear that there are too many variables for any manufacturer to actually accomplish the goals proposed. Imagine presenting this many variables to a group of mathematicians and asking them, "What is the likelihood that we will ever be able to successfully combine the vitamins and minerals per the recommendations?" They would probably laugh at the improbability of ever finding a solution. It is simpler to bite into an apple than to reconstruct one.

Synergy

One of the best known synergistic relationships is the one between vitamin C and vitamin E, and it is probably representative of countless, as yet unknown relationships that exist between nutrients. Vitamin C and E have similar capacities to neutralize free radicals, but go about their work in completely different areas of the cell. Vitamin C is water-soluble and does its work in the aqueous solution of the cell, whereas vitamin E is fat-soluble and does its work on membranes that are made up of fatty acids. Now, here comes an example of a relationship made in heaven: when vitamin E on the surface of a membrane becomes a radical itself after neutralizing a lipid peroxide molecule, vitamin C in the surrounding solution can regenerate that vitamin E radical. This is exactly how the vitamin E molecules found on fatty LDL particles work in concert with the vitamin C molecules in the surrounding blood to protect the blood serum LDL from being oxidized. Furthermore, synergistic protection provided by these two vitamins together appears to be *greater* than the *sum* of the protective roles of each in preventing oxidative damage (Niki et al., 1995). We are just beginning to understand how different antioxidants work together to provide greater protection. Such synergistic relationships suggest that it may be some time before vitamin and mineral supplements will be able to duplicate Mother Nature.

Isomers

An isomer is one of several possible three-dimensional configurations of the atoms of a molecule; isomers may be mirror images of the same compound. Nature seems to have a preference for one of the mirror images over the other. When nutrients are chemically manufactured, the body only recognizes one preferred isomer, while the other isomer is of no use to the body. When chemicals are ingested and not utilized, such as these unused isomers, it takes a toll on the body, since various tissues now have to get involved in the disposal of these unused chemicals. This is an inherent problem with synthetic nutrients.

Multiple components of a nutrient

In addition to the isomer problem, vitamin supplements also neglect to differentiate between the various components that make up a vitamin. Let's consider vitamin E. It's made up of at least eight components that have been isolated: four tocopherols and four tocotrienols. However, most supplements only contain one component of vitamin E, alpha-tocopherol, and this is usually synthetically manufactured. Again, synthesizing alpha-tocopherol would produce isomers that would be different from those found in nature (Papas, 1999). So, a vitamin E supplement is necessarily inferior in several important ways:

- It doesn't contain all of the eight known components of vitamin E.
- Half of the one component it is likely to have is in the

wrong isomer form for the body to utilize.
- It may not contain any components or crucial cofactors of vitamin E that may still be isolated in the future.

Clearly, complete vitamin E from food sources or whole food based concentrates is preferable to isolated supplementation. Case in point: the function of gamma-tocopherol. The microflora that naturally live in the bowel can generate hydroxyl free radicals at a rate corresponding to that produced by 10,000 rads of gamma radiation per day (Babbs and Steiner, 1990). Gamma tocopherol is the principle antioxidant in colon tissue that fights this free radical production (Stone and Papas, 1997). Now, next time you go to buy vitamin E, read the label carefully to see if the manufacturer tells you whether you are getting all eight components in their desired isomers as found in whole food.

Localization

We're also just beginning to appreciate how different antioxidants, when ingested from whole foods, are found in higher concentrations in different tissues. We've already discussed that gamma-tocopherol tends to localize in the colon. Other examples exist in the carotenoid family of antioxidants: lycopenes like to localize in the skin and prostate gland, whereas beta-carotene is found in many places in the body; luteins and zeaxanthins also localize in different tissues. When these nutrients are ingested in whole food form, research shows that the proper localization of each antioxidant occurs. Whereas, supplementation with isolated components can lead to too much accumulation in one tissue and not enough in others (Micozzi et al., 1992; Stone and Papas, 1997; Wise et al., 1996). It's as if the antioxidants ingested from whole food come with first class postage and a complete delivery address, whereas vitamin supplements are delivered with bulk postage to "current resident."

A word about tests that determine deficiencies

I often hear people say that they have been tested for specific vitamin or mineral deficiencies, such as low levels of zinc or magnesium or vitamin C, and that they have begun taking supplements based solely on the results of such testing. This approach truly perplexes me. If there are deficiencies, then it is because entire food groups are missing from one's diet. Supplementation based on the results of such testing is part and parcel of the big vitamin hoax. For instance, if we eat an orange, do we tell the body: "Don't absorb the bioflavinoids, but go ahead and absorb the vitamin C"? No, we either eat the orange or don't eat the orange. So, if the test includes both vitamin C and bioflavinoids, then we'll see that we're missing both, especially since it turns out that bioflavinoids are necessary for vitamin C absorption. If the test does not look for a bioflavinoid deficiency, then we'll only learn about the vitamin C deficiency, be content to buy a vitamin C pill, and never even know that we're lacking the bioflavinoids required to assimilate the vitamin C. What you don't know can hurt you.

Tests for specific nutrient deficiencies only serve to make supplements seem more legitimate, but they are not founded in logic. If a person is anemic, she can't expect a "cure" by taking an iron supplement, because iron is probably not the only thing that's missing in her diet. In general, she

Nutrient tested as deficient	Additional nutrients known to be needed for assimilation
Vitamin A	Choline, essential fatty acids, zinc, vitamins C, D and E
Vitamin B Complex	Calcium, vitamins C and E
Vitamin B₁(thiamine)	Manganese, vitamin B complex, vitamins C and E
Vitamin B₂ (riboflavin)	Vitamin B complex, vitamin C
Vitamin B₃ (niacin)	Vitamin B complex, vitamin C
Vitamin B₅ (pantothenic acid)	Vitamin B complex, vitamin A, C and E
Vitamin B₆ (pyridoxine)	Potassium, vitamin B complex, vitamin C
Biotin	Folic acid, vitamin B complex, pantothenic acid, vitamin B₁₂, vitamin C
Choline	Vitamin B complex, vitamin B₁₂, folic acid, inositol
Inositol	Vitamin B complex, vitamin C
Para-aminobenzoic acid	Vitamin B complex, folic acid, vitamin C
Vitamin C	Bioflavonoids, calcium, magnesium
Vitamin D	Calcium, choline, essential fatty acids, phosphorus, vitamins A and C
Vitamin E	Essential fatty acids, manganese, selenium, vitamin A, vitamin B₁, inositol, vitamin C
Essential fatty acids	Vitamins A, C, D and E
Calcium	Boron, essential fatty acids, lysine, magnesium, manganese, phosphorus, vitamins A, C, D and E
Copper	Cobalt, folic acid, iron, zinc
Iodine	Iron, manganese, phosphorus
Magnesium	Calcium, phosphorus, potassium, vitamin B₆, vitamin C and D
Manganese	Calcium, iron, vitamin B complex, vitamin E
Phosphorus	Calcium, iron, manganese, sodium, vitamin B₆
Silicon	Iron, phosphorus
Sodium	Calcium, potassium, sulfur, vitamin D
Sulfur	Potassium, vitamin B₁, vitamin B₅, biotin
Zinc	Calcium, copper, phosphorus, vitamin B₆

Figure 10. Interactions between nutrients (Balch and Balch, 1997)

needs to eat more protein and let her body do the rest.

In *Figure 10*, we see a list of some of the known inter-actions between nutrients in terms of absorption or assimi-lation. Let me say that this table represents only the tip of the iceberg and the state of our knowledge back in 1997.

Even though we still don't have all of the data necessary to create a table showing a complete set of interactions, we can already see that isolated vitamin and mineral supple-ments would leave big gaps in our overall nutritional requirements. The following illustration serves as a good demonstration of the problem.

What your body sees with vitamin pills:

T k r ght t th H ds n Str t G t th f rst tr ff c l ght nd st y n l ft l n t m k l ft n M ntg m r y Blvd P ss thr st p s gns nd f ll w c rv d r d p th h ll t th f rth st p s gn. M k r ght n M ch g n Str t.

What your body sees with whole food:

Take a right at the Hudson Street. Go to the first traffic light and stay in left lane to make a left on Montgomery Blvd. Pass three stop signs and follow curved road up the hill to the fourth stop sign. Make a right on Michigan Street.

Well, how would you like to look at your world? I think it's clear that if we want to get where we're going, we'd better be able to read the directions! Obviously, whole foods and whole food based concentrates help us to stay on the right track.

Claims and quality control

We have become a nation of label-readers. We pride ourselves on knowing what we are putting into our bodies. But sometimes what it says on the label or in the ad and what is actually contained in the product are two very different things. Also, there are technical challenges in the production of supplements that go above and beyond any lack of regulation in the supplement industry. Many independent studies show that supplements:

- often fall short of the nutrients they say that they have on the label
- are marketed using unsubstantiated claims
- lack bioavailability data
- lack sufficient testing

There are not enough studies being done in the industry to know if vitamin supplementation is even doing any good. (Ames, 1999; Hoag et al., 1997; Newman et al., 1987). The obvious, and somewhat alarming, flip side to this is that we don't have enough data to know all the ways in which such isolated supplementation may be causing harm. Even when there is an attempt to show research, it is usually what is called "structure/function" research. What this means is that a manufacturer will advertise that "nutrient such and such" is known to be beneficial to our health. Then they will make available scientific papers on "nutrient such and such" for consumers to read. Then they will claim that because their product has "nutrient such and such" in it, it is a product that should give you the same results as seen in the research.

There is a major flaw in this structure/function approach: claims actually say nothing about whether the product being sold does any good, because the product itself doesn't have credible independent data to back it up. The FDA is now trying to come up with guidelines for structure/function claims. Nevertheless, these claims are how most supplements get sold; and, with powerful industry lobbies in Washington, they will probably continue to contribute, in some form or other, to the great vitamin hoax.

I hope that it's now clearer than ever that we need to change our diets instead of relying on isolated supplements. Taking isolated supplements to make up for deficiencies from poor food choices will only perpetuate the toxic food environment aspect of the Default Health Program. When I think of the challenge facing anyone who hopes to manufacture the ultimate supplement from isolated nutrients, I am reminded of the nursery rhyme:

Humpty Dumpty sat on a wall.
Humpty Dumpty had a great fall.
All the king's horses and all the king's men
Couldn't put Humpty together again!

A program for optimal health has no place for the unanswered questions and technical difficulties associated with isolated supplements. Fortunately, there is no need for isolated supplements when the diet provides nutrients from appropriate food sources. Finally, if it's difficult to take in a large variety of raw vegetables and fruits consistently at every meal, then whole food based supplements can be an extremely beneficial part of the equation for optimal health.

We've already looked at Juice Plus+®, and we'll talk more about whole food based supplementation as we wend our way along the path *From Here to Longevity.*

10

Ancient Pyramids

Until now, our discussion has focussed mostly on nutrients that don't provide any calories. These are generally called micronutrients. Antioxidants, minerals, phytochemicals, and vitamins come under the heading of micronutrients. As we've learned, micronutrients protect molecules from free-radical damage, and act as cofactors that make chemical reactions in the body proceed more efficiently. In other words, they protect and serve cells at the molecular level.

Now it's time to meet the other half of the diet puzzle—macronutrients. Unlike *micro*nutrients, *macro*nutrients *do* have caloric value. They serve as the building blocks for important chemicals in the body, and they operate on a broader level than micronutrients. *Macro*nutrients are primarily needed for overall energy, proper hormonal function, and tissue maintenance and repair. As we've discussed, there are hundreds of micronutrients, and new ones are being discovered all the time. In all probability, there are perhaps several thousand micronutrients that will eventually be found in our food. In contrast, macronutrients are fewer in number, three to be exact—proteins, fats and carbohydrates; and there's a high probability that new macronutrients will never be discovered.

Even though we've known about these three macronutrients for quite some time now, they remain a subject of debate. Currently, a hot topic in the field of nutrition is the proportion in which these three should be consumed. A subtopic of the controversy concerns which kinds of proteins, fats, or carbohydrates best serve our health. Here, it becomes more important than ever to distinguish between micronutrients and macronutrients, since the quality of the three macronutrients has a lot to do with the amount of micronutrients that each contains. For example, a piece of bread and a piece of carrot are both carbohydrates, but the carrot has many more micronutrients, making it a superior choice of carbohydrate when it comes to nutritive value.

Over the years since their discovery, a simplistic view of macronutrients has emerged. This oversimplification of macronutrients includes the following ideas:

- If you want to lose weight, simply reduce your caloric intake.
- The fat that you eat becomes the fat that you end up wearing on your body.
- Only athletes need to eat a lot of protein; the rest of us could do with less.
- We should eat lots of grains for energy.

In reality, the macronutrients that we eat determine which hormones get triggered and this, in turn, affects blood sugar, body fat and lean mass. In other words, we can't just tally up the number of grams of proteins, fats and carbohydrates we had at the end of the day; nor can we simply tally up the number of total calories consumed. At each meal, we must consider the effect of that meal on our hormones. This is not the usual relationship people have with the food that they eat. In this chapter, I'll discuss our current relationship to macronutrients in the Default Health Program. I'll also point out how hormones are affected by food. This will lay the groundwork for the next chapter, where I'll dispel some common myths about food.

In response to the oversimplified views about macronutrients, experts have offered us various explanations with such best-selling titles as:

- *Fit for Life* by Harvey and Marilyn Diamond (Warner Books, 1985)
- *Diet for a New America* by John Robbins (Stillpoint Publishing, 1987)
- *Dr. Atkins' New Diet Revolution* by Robert C. Atkins, M.D. (Avon Books, 1992)
- *Enter the Zone* by Barry Sears, Ph.D. (Harper Collins, 1995)
- *Eat Right For Your Type* by Dr. Peter J. D'Adamo (Putnam, 1997)
- *Eat, Drink and Be Healthy* by Dr. Walter C. Willett (Simon and Schuster, 2001)

These books cover such important topics as:

- not mixing the three macronutrients in the same meal
- choosing macronutrients according to blood type or body type

- being in "the Zone"
- becoming a vegetarian
- *not* becoming a vegetarian

Even after all these years of study and research, we're all still grappling with a basic understanding of macronutrients. While each new book seems to enlighten us further, no one is the ultimate authority on this topic. However, as we gather more and more information, these authors, as well as other independent sources, are finally coming to similar conclusions. So let's talk about this broader picture of macronutrients that is emerging out of these converging viewpoints.

One of the biggest pieces of the puzzle that most experts now agree on is the importance of avoiding processed foods. These foods often advertise the words "fat-free" and "cholesterol-free." Such advertising "buzz" words thrive on the current mythology around food. Processed foods are, in fact, made up of proteins, fats and carbohydrates; but the quality of these macronutrients is so damaged that it's perhaps more accurate to call them "anti-nutrients." The real culprits, as we'll discover in *Chapter Eleven*, are two particular anti-nutrients—processed sugars and damaged fats. Once we can eliminate these two culprits, we'll see that eating right is really quite simple.

First, it's important to understand how our bodies and our very quality of life depend upon the foods we eat. Let's start by looking at the table on the following page that lists just some of the functions that are affected by the macronutrients we choose:

Function	Regulation of Function
Energy level	Macronutrients provide the calories we need to burn for energy.
Mood	Macronutrients regulate "emotion hormones," such as endorphins and serotonin.
Stress response	Macronutrients regulate "stress hormones," such as cortisol; they also regulate "blood sugar hormones," such as insulin and glucagons, which can ultimately affect the "stress hormones."
Body composition	Macronutrients affect how much lean tissue (the more we have, the better) and how much body fat we have (another function of "blood sugar hormones").
Sex-related functions	Macronutrients affect hot flashes, normal menstruation, infertility, sex drive, virility, and puberty and growth in children; these functions are regulated by the "sex hormones" such as androgen, progesterone, estrogen and growth hormone.

In fact, optimal health can be achieved only when:

- the body has the energy it needs to function
- the important hormones that regulate emotions, stress response, sexual function, and blood sugar are all present in adequate amounts and, most importantly, in balance with one another

This balance is in fact so crucial that it has a special name: homeostasis. Homeostasis is a state in which all of the interdependent chemicals in the body are in a physiological balance that is appropriate for the time of day and a person's sex, age, weight, activity level and overall health.

Homeostasis is when you feel good because all the chemicals in your body are *naturally* in balance, without drugs or stimulants. Hormone levels will fluctuate within a safe range over the course of a day (see *Figure 11* below). It's when these hormones go out of the safe zone that the disease process can take over.

When the body doesn't get the right amount of proteins, fats, or carbohydrates, the hormones in the body fall out of homeostasis. This can have profound implications for short- and long-term health. How do we respond when these hormones fall out of homeostasis? All too often we go for a quick fix instead of providing the body with what it's really looking for—proper rest, proper exercise and a balanced diet of micronutrient-rich proteins, fats and carbohydrates. For instance, if we feel tired and sluggish, we may choose to have a cup of coffee or some other stimulant or drug, or a baked goodie. We choose these foods or stimulants because they release certain "emotion hormones," such as serotonin, which make us feel good immediately.

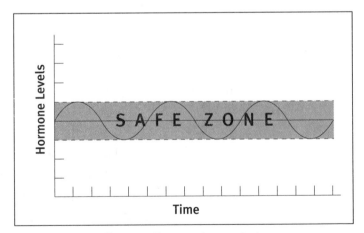

Figure 11. Hormone homeostasis

However, this feeling doesn't last very long. We hear, "Drink more coffee!" or "Have a glass of wine!" when what the body is really trying to tell us is that it needs a balanced meal—or maybe a nap or a good workout. We've misread the body's signal, and unfortunately, stimulants and drugs aren't going to help us build muscle tissue, or repair the daily damage to our enzymes. In fact, the *body* is never trying to tell us, "Hey, I need to repair this cell here, so please get me some more nicotine or caffeine or alcohol or sugar!" But that doesn't mean that we don't hear the *brain* saying, "Get me some more nicotine or caffeine or alcohol or a sugar!" Because these substances release emotion hormones right away, we can easily find ourselves addicted to them.

You may be thinking, "I haven't been in an accident or broken a bone. Why should I be worrying about repairing tissue?" You don't need to have sustained some sort of injury for this to be a priority. Every day, the body needs to devote some time and energy to the repair and rebuilding of enzymes and other components of lean tissue. Most of this happens at night. So, what you eat during the day not only provides you with the energy for your day's activities, but also supplies your body with the materials it needs to build and make repairs at night.

Most human beings operate from the standpoint that it's OK to not be super strict with eating right, managing stress and exercising. "Someday, when I get my money, love life and time management all worked out, I'll start exercising and eating better." Reality check. Now hear this! The effects of food, drug and stimulant intake on hormone homeostasis are regulated by a principle not unlike the Law of Gravity. Gravity is *always* there for us to deal with. Whenever you drop something, it *always* heads toward the ground. Any time you jump into the air, you'll *always* have to come back down to the earth. Now, this doesn't mean that you can never eat dessert. Just know that the "Laws of the Body" still apply—always have, always will. There is no negotiating with the "Laws of the Body," just as there is no negotiating with the Law of Gravity. *We will finally be able to manage our health when we make choices that respect and work consciously with the strict natural laws that govern how the body can operate.* As a good friend once said in a moment of epiphany, "I thought for sure that I could eat a little extra, exercise now and then, and not gain weight. Like, wow, how did this happen to me? I thought that the rules didn't apply all the time." By the time you've finished reading this book, you'll have the critical information you need to develop a powerful relationship with the laws that govern the body.

For instance, when the body runs low on the "emotion hormone" serotonin, and we don't respond by eating the real food that the body needs in order to replenish its supply of serotonin, we're going to find ourselves reaching for an addictive stimulant. Over time we may even feel that we need to increase our intake of stimulants in an attempt to get the same "high" we experienced the last time.

The chemical that most of us are addicted to in food is sugar. William Dufty, author of *Sugar Blues* (Warner Books, 1976), writes of his experience as he committed himself to removing all the processed sugar in his diet:

I threw all the sugar out of my kitchen. Then I threw out everything that had sugar in it, cereals, and canned fruit, soups and bread. Since I had never really read any labels carefully, I was shocked to find the shelves were soon empty. So was the refrigerator.... I knew enough about junkies to recognize reluctantly my kinship with them. After all, heroin is nothing but a chemical. They take the juice of the poppy...refine it into opium...refine it to morphine and finally to heroin. Sugar is nothing but a chemical. They take the juice of the cane or the beet...refine it to molasses...refine it to brown sugar and finally to strange white crystals.

While we can expect headaches and other symptoms of detoxification when we try to kick the processed sugar habit, the alternative is to continue to place our bodies at risk for all of the other ailments that comprise the Default Health Program.

Like other neurotransmitters (chemicals in the brain that are responsible for communication), serotonin is very expensive for the body to manufacture in terms of raw materials and energy. It requires amino acids, especially tryptophan, for synthesis and these amino acids are supplied by a diet that includes adequate protein, especially animal protein. This hefty price tag encourages the body to recycle serotonin as much as it can before it has to make a new batch.

Drug companies have found a way to take advantage of the body's recycling of serotonin. Some antidepressant drugs, such as Prozac®, essentially shut down the recycling system. This, in turn, allows serotonin to hang around longer for your nerve cells, which gives you a short-term gain of feeling happy. Sounds nice, right? The problem is that, just like sugar, antidepressants can be addictive as well. There have been several lawsuits brought against GlaxoSmithKline, the makers of the second most popular antidepressant, Paxil®. The most recent lawsuit contends that the company hid Paxil's addictive nature. On August 26, 2001, *The Seattle Times* reported that

> ...a lawsuit was filed...on behalf of 35 people around the country who say they suffered symptoms ranging from electric-like shocks to suicidal thoughts after discontinuing use of the drug. The lawsuit...says GlaxoSmithKline PLC concealed the possibility of physical and psychological withdrawal symptoms from the drug. It alleges fraud, deceit, negligence, liability and breach of warranty (The Seattle Times, 2001).

Underlying any apparent success or failure with antidepressants is the fact that these drugs may only be masking symptoms. Symptoms are the messages the body sends us to tell us something is wrong. Any discomfort, be it physical or emotional, is a signal of the body falling out of homeostasis. Sometimes a temporary loss of equilibrium is appropriate, as during grief over the loss of a loved one or in the preparation for a new challenge. Let me be clear that what I'm referring to here is the ongoing state of not being in homeostasis as result of diet and lifestyle, which is so much a part of the Default Health Program.

Whether a state of depression were being handled by a drug or not, the drug would still not be addressing the more fundamental problem of an imbalance of hormones in the body. As a result, other disease processes would continue to progress and the drug would allow a person to ignore the symptoms. I'm not saying that it's wrong to use antidepressants. What I *am* saying is that it's important to remember that the body is still out of balance—even when the symptoms are being managed.

Another problem with depression is that many people self-prescribe so-called "natural" alternatives like St. John's Wort. Even if they call or visit a clinic or general practitioner, they may walk out with a prescription without undergoing a thorough examination or an exhaustive interview. No one should go on antidepressants without first checking such basic things as blood sugar, thyroid levels, blood pressure, and diet. Regardless of the diagnosis or the drug treatment, we still want to give the body the building blocks it needs to make not only sufficient serotonin, but all of the other important hormones as well.

I also don't want to give the impression that if a person is shown by preliminary testing to have abnormal thyroid levels, then thyroid medications are necessarily more appropriate. When a person is malnourished, the body protects itself by decreasing thyroid hormone production, since normal amounts of thyroid would further break down body tissue for protein utilization. The symptoms of hypothyroidism and malnutrition are similar: fatigue, inability to generate body heat, hair loss, weight gain, dry skin and constipation. Treating malnutrition with either antidepressants

Hormone Homeostasis:
Common Contributing Factors for Chemical Imbalance

Sugar hormones Insulin and Glucagon	1. Diet high in processed carbohydrates (breads, pastas, crackers, etc.) 2. Diet high in bad fats (trans, oxidized, hydrogenated) 3. Low-fat diet 4. Low protein diet 5. Lack of exercise 6. Diet lacking in vegetables and fruits
Stress hormones Glucocorticoids Epinephrine Norepinephrine	1. Prenatal conditions 2. Infant care 3. Prolonged stress 4. Lack of exercise 5. Diet lacking vegetables and fruits
Emotion hormones Serotonin Dopamine	1. Lack of exercise 2. Emotional stress 3. Diet lacking B vitamins, calcium, magnesium, tryptophan 4. Vegan diets 5. Chemical stimulants (alcohol, caffeine, tobacco, diet pills, ma huang, etc.)
Sex hormones Estrogen Progesterone Androgen Testosterone	1. Prenatal conditions 2. Low-fat diet 3. Organic toxins (heated plastics)

or thyroid medication causes a person's general health to further deteriorate. Again, they mask the deeper, underlying problem and interfere with the body's normal mechanisms that are designed to try to protect it during periods of malnutrition (Schwarzbein and Deville, 1999).

From looking at the first table, you can appreciate how

Hormone Homeostasis:
Contributing Factors for Healing and Longevity

Sugar hormones
Insulin and
Glucagon
	1. Fiber-rich carbohydrates
	   (vegetables and fruits)
	2. Sufficient protein
	3. Sufficient poly-unsaturated fats
	   (uncooked)
	4. Moderate exercise

Stress hormones
Glucocorticoids
Epinephrine
Norepinephrine
	1. Meditation
	2. Moderate exercise
	3. Yoga and other stress-releasing activities
	4. Balanced diet of fiber rich carbohdrates
	   (vegetables and fruits), protein and
	   poly-unsaturated fats
	5. Healthy relationships with family and
	   friends

Emotion hormones
Serotonin
Dopamine
	1. Balanced diet of fiber rich carbohydrates
	   (vegetables and fruits), protein and
	   poly-unsaturated fats
	2. Exercise

Sex hormones Estrogen Progesterone Androgen Testosterone	1. Hormone replacement therapy 2. Diet rich in essential fatty acids

various aspects of the Default Health Program throw hormones out of balance. The second table shows you how much control you really have to reestablish hormone homeostasis. But when should you pay attention to this list, and what are the symptoms of hormone imbalance? Consider that other than the random injury or infectious disease, most chronic health complaints may be at least partly, if not totally attributed to hormone imbalance. Insomnia, indigestion, bloating, gout, ulcers, skin diseases, lack of concentration, irritability, headaches, chronic aches and pains, diabetes, frequent colds, infertility, impotence, depression and heart disease are just some of the manifestations of hormone imbalance. Further consider that these maladies are just ways of getting our attention. The body is screaming, "Wake up! For crying out loud, eat right, exercise and mellow out!"

So why don't we do it? First, once we've sent the body into an addictive cycle, it takes time for it to use food to bring these hormone levels back to homeostasis. It takes only minutes for a drug to conceal a symptom, but it takes months for food to heal the body. If you were to change your diet in order to lose weight, you'd expect to wait at least a few weeks before results were visible. Hopefully, you'd trust that you were going to get results, even if you couldn't see them yet. The same is true when you make the dietary changes necessary for the body to return to homeostasis. You won't wake up the very next morning with all of your hormones and body processes functioning perfectly. It will take some time before dramatic results are visible. Your job is to stick with those lifestyle changes and exercise your patience, while your body gets on with its task of healing itself. When you're tempted to give up, just remember—there's no place like homeostasis!

In addition to this personal challenge of being patient, there are two more reasons why we, as a society, have lost faith in the power of food. One is the availability and convenience of junk foods as compared to the relative lack of availability and perceived inconvenience of whole food. Another is that people are often misguided about what whole food is. We've already determined that the toxic food environment is bad for our genes. Unfortunately, more often than not, traditional social gatherings promote detrimental eating habits. Whether we're meeting friends for coffee or drinks, attending a picnic, party or potluck, or going out to dinner, it can be uncomfortable to draw attention to ourselves by saying "No" to the foods and drinks that other people are having. Thus, one of the foundations on which the Default Health Program is built is what I call the Junk Food Pyramid. Without it, the Default Health Program could never have gained momentum. Major health problems begin the moment we start eating processed food laden with damaged fats and sugar.

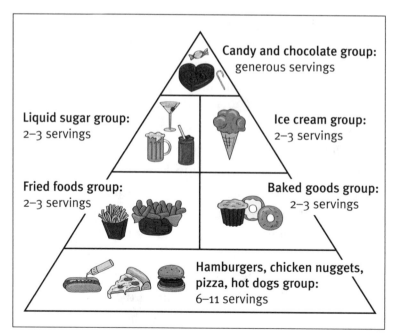

Figure 12. The Junk Food Pyramid

Typically, a person will follow this junk food regimen until the symptoms of disease become too uncomfortable. Then it's time for a trip to the doctor, who writes a prescription. We've already discussed the pitfalls of pharmaceuticals. If the doctor has your long-term interest at heart, he or she may suggest that you try to change your lifestyle as well.

Part of that recommendation would be to have you give up the Junk Food Pyramid, and start eating according to the USDA Food Guide Pyramid—a low fat, low cholesterol, high carbohydrate diet. If you take heed of your doctor's advice, you may get some short-term benefits. Then, eventually, your health will deteriorate again and you'll think it's because you're just getting older or that you just lack will power. We're so used to blaming ourselves that we don't question the USDA Food Guide Pyramid; and yet, questioning the USDA Food Guide Pyramid is exactly what I'm suggesting. First of all, scientists didn't come up with the USDA Food Guide Pyramid. The government came up with the USDA Food Guide Pyramid. And I suspect that lobbyists representing different food industries probably had something to do with the selection of these various food groups and their respective positions. After all, it is the *United States Department of Agriculture* Food Guide Pyramid, not the National Institutes of Health or the National Academy of Sciences Food Pyramid.

In fact, Dr. Walter C. Willett, the chairman of the Department of Nutrition at the Harvard School of Public Health and a professor of medicine at the Harvard Medical School, has spoken out against the USDA Food Guide

Pyramid in his book, *Eat, Drink and Be Healthy* (Simon & Schuster Source, 2001). He, too, believes that the creation of the USDA Food Guide Pyramid was motivated more by certain food industries than by valid scientific research. According to Dr. Willett, not only is it not backed by valid research, it also isn't making much of a contribution to most people's lives either. In 1993, when I first started to become concerned about my weight, I also started to eat according to the USDA Food Guide Pyramid. Eating pasta and rice, while avoiding fat, just made me get fatter. And I know I'm not alone in this.

The Federal Government claims that it created this USDA Food Guide Pyramid in an attempt to reduce the risk of major chronic disease (with the added benefit of pro-

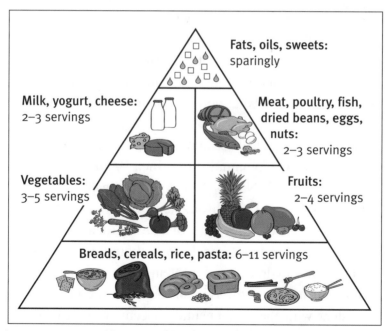

Figure 13. USDA Food Guide Pyramid

moting agriculture). Nonetheless, there a lack of scientific data that supports adhering to these recommendations.

Government and medical experts have been generally recommending a diet low in fat and high in carbohydrates, with the thought that a low-fat diet will reduce the risk of heart disease, obesity, diabetes and the like. It turns out that this is too simplistic an approach.

One study did show a weak association between adherence to this guide and the risk of major chronic disease (McCullough et al., 2000). This weak association is not surprising to me. Whenever we stop to notice what we are eating and follow any kind of a restricted diet—even if it's the Grapefruit Juice diet—there's always the possibility that something good might happen. People usually get some results, even if it's for no other reason than that paying attention a little bit is better than not paying attention at all. That is, any plan at all is slightly better than the Junk Food Pyramid. But when it comes to achieving optimal health, not any old "watch what you eat" plan will do.

Recently, I came across another book—*The Schwarzbein Principle* (Health Communications Inc., 1999) by Dr. Diana Schwarzbein and Nancy Deville—that really made an impression on me. Dr. Schwarzbein's medical practice has included extensive work with diabetes patients. Her case studies confirm my own conclusions about the proportions of fats, carbohydrates and proteins that we should be eating. Furthermore, the type of medicine she practices is consistent with the fundamental concepts of biochemistry and physiology. According to Dr. Schwarzbein's experience,

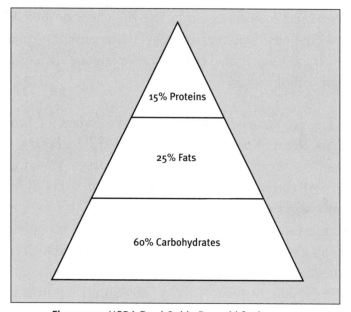

Figure 14a. USDA Food Guide Pyramid for humans

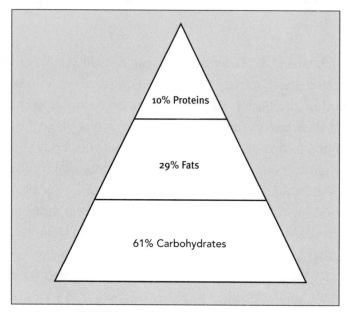

Figure 14b. USDA Food Guide Pyramid for fattening cattle

telling heart patients to eat by the guidelines of the USDA Food Guide Pyramid has often led to the onset of diabetes. Also, it has exacerbated conditions for anyone already diagnosed with diabetes.

The recommendation to eat 6-11 servings of breads, cereals, rice and pasta—the bulk of the USDA Food Guide Pyramid—is really a recommendation to eat 6-11 servings of sugar. All carbohydrates get broken down in the body to the simple sugar called "glucose," whether they started out as pasta, bread, crackers, pretzels, chips, rice or cereal. So, it doesn't have to taste sweet to be sugar; and too much sugar in the diet leads to insulin-related health challenges, such as diabetes and obesity. This is not surprising when we observe that the proportions of proteins, fats and carbohydrates on the USDA Food Guide Pyramid are alarmingly similar to the USDA guidelines for fattening cattle and other live stock.

Consider that every time you eat, a small sample of your digested meal moves across the intestinal wall into the blood of the portal vein and then travels to the liver. The liver then has to make intelligent decisions about how to respond to this meal you have just given your body. One of its primary concerns is supplying the right amount of sugar to your brain. So if you eat too much sugar, it secretes the "blood sugar hormone" insulin in order to try to bring sugar levels back into homeostasis. The bottom line is that whether you follow the Junk Food Pyramid or the USDA Food Guide Pyramid, both prescribe a diet high in sugar content, and adherence to either diet will lead to an ongoing rise in insulin levels. In other words, both diets are ultimately highly detrimental to the body.

Prolonged high levels of insulin can lead to:

Acne
Addictions
Asthma
Cancer
Delayed puberty
Depression
Eating disorders
Excessive weight gain
Heartburn or other gastrointestinal disorders
Heart disease
High cholesterol and triglyceride levels
Infertility
Insomnia and fatigue
Insulin resistance leading to Type II diabetes
Irritable bowel syndrome
Low estrogen
Migraine headaches
Osteoporosis

On the other hand, if you don't eat enough sugar, then you'll secrete the "blood sugar hormone" glucagon, which will, in turn, start to release stored sugar in order to serve the brain. Once the body runs out of its limited amount of stored sugar, it turns to breaking down protein matter and converting that to sugar for energy. This is just what happens in people who skip breakfast. No matter what we eat or don't eat, the body always has essential metabolic needs. For instance, it needs carbohydrates as fuel for the brain, fats for maintaining body temperature, and proteins for making enzymes and antibodies. So, if you don't eat breakfast after a night of fasting, the body is forced to break down its own tissue in order to supply its most urgent necessities for macronutrients. Breakfast-skippers actually end up eating themselves for breakfast.

Eating up your own body might sound like the way to lose weight, but in fact it produces the reverse effect. Both for our appearance and for our health, we need to maintain as much lean body mass as possible and to minimize body fat. What is lean body mass? It is your muscles, organs, bones, skin, ligaments and basically anything else that isn't fatty tissue. The more you have of it, the healthier you'll be, and, because your metabolic rate will be higher with more lean mass, the easier you'll lose any excess fat.

The real trick would be to eat such balanced meals throughout the day that the ratio of insulin to glucagon would allow the body to be in homeostasis. This is a concept that Barry Sears hit upon in his book *Enter the Zone*, and one that many other books, including *The Schwarzbein Principle*, have since refined. *It is ironic that the evolution of our knowledge about nutrition is directing us back to the Stone Age diet of our ancestors.* In order to re-create the optimal diet, we must realize that not all fats, proteins and carbohydrates are created equal. Furthermore, the calories from each of these sources are not equal either.

I'll discuss all of this in the next chapter, but what I want to do most at this juncture is give away the punch line first. *The secret to optimal health is to eat micronutrient-rich macronutrients in a balance that promotes hormone home-ostasis.* This promotes the building and repairing of lean body mass, rather than the building of body fat and the tearing down of lean body mass.

I'm now going to make some bold and revolutionary statements that could challenge your most deeply held beliefs about food and nutrition. You may even question my sanity, but just stay with me at least until the next chapter when all will become clearer.

Advising people to eat micronutrient-rich macronutrients in such proportion that the insulin to glucagons ratio stays in balance may seem logical enough. Nevertheless, eating this way means eating Mother Nature's food with all its macronutrients intact, including things like cholesterol and saturated fat. Just try telling medical doctors that they should advise their patients *not* to avoid saturated fats or cholesterol, and they'll tell you that you've lost your mind. Why? For years, most doctors have been recommending skim or reduced-fat milk and yogurt; they are convinced that low-fat foods are best for their patients. But *whole* food actually means whole milk or regular yogurt, instead of the skim or reduced-fat versions, even though these low-fat foods are what is usually advised and what most people still believe to be a better choice. Whole food also means vegetables and fruits, not fragmented vitamin supplements, or fruit juices where the fiber has been removed and all that remains are sugar and a handful of vitamins. Even freshly made juices are generally missing the fiber that balances the sugar content, and drinking them causes the body to secrete too much insulin. Whole food means butter, not margarine.

Whole food means omelets or scrambled eggs made with whole, organic eggs, not just egg whites. Thus, whole food—including whole food concentrates, as found in Juice Plus+®; and other nutraceuticals, such as omega-3 fatty acid supplements—supports the root system of the Longevity Tree (*Figure 26*, page 340) by approaching health from the perspective of prevention of disease in every cell of the body.

The controversy doesn't end with skim milk vs. whole milk. We're also being asked to consider soy milk, rice milk and other milk substitutes. But do we really need them? Some people have an intolerance to milk. Dark circles around the eyes often indicate an allergic reaction to dairy. Others have a hard time digesting the milk sugar called "lactose." If you don't have either problem, then you could drink it; although I would advise you to always buy organic, whole milk and, if possible, to choose from local dairies.

I know that most people who are health-conscious tend to avoid milk. I myself avoided it for years. But, taking a closer look, I couldn't convince myself that there was really any solid foundation to the bad reputation that milk has been getting. In fact, whole milk is a balanced source of complete protein, low-glycemic index carbohydrates, calcium and important fats. While some cannot tolerate milk, others seem to thrive on it. And a glass of warm milk can be a wonderful sleep-enhancer. I'm always in favor of a good night's rest.

The next point about milk substitutes is that nutritionally speaking, they're really not milk substitutes at all, since they are plant-based. Most of them are high in carbohydrates and low in protein. Rice milk is also low in fat. You should not choose a product that has no fiber and more than 10 grams of carbohydrates per serving (usually 1 cup). I recommend the organic, unsweetened soy milk brands that have only 5–9 grams of carbohydrates, as well as 3–4 grams of fiber. These brands also tend to have a good amount of protein and fat. Do not choose low-fat or vanilla flavored or otherwise sweetened varieties.

The third point is that while soy milk is a good idea for women over 30 years of age, there is some controversy as to whether men or children should drink it at all. Some people go "soy crazy" and that's not smart for anyone. Soy milk is not a good idea for pregnant or lactating women and soy formulas are not a good idea for infants and toddlers. The same plant hormones that may serve as beneficial to women, may not be a good idea for men and young children, especially in excess.

There is also an ongoing disagreement about the right balance of macronutrients. A balance of proteins, carbohydrates and fats means a breakfast of two eggs, an apple and a cup of yogurt made from whole milk; balance does not mean a bowl of non-fat cereal (whole grain or processed) with non-fat milk and a glass of orange juice. The non-fat breakfast is what is known as a carbohydrate-intense meal. Such a meal is guaranteed to increase insulin levels. It resembles the typical vegetarian meal that is also thought to be healthy: one cup of brown rice and one cup of kidney beans, which weighs in at 20 grams of protein and 90 grams of carbohydrates. Neither the non-fat breakfast nor the vegetarian meal is a contender; the body never needs that many carbohydrates in one meal! In fact, 30 grams is plenty; and, if you're trying to lose body fat, you might even choose to limit each meal to 15 grams of carbohydrates.

Depending on where you are in your journey toward longevity, you may be shocked or surprised at this juncture. I warned you that you might end up questioning my sanity. Yet, there is a voice inside you quietly saying, "Hmm, this makes some sense; but it's contrary to what my doctor said, or what I read, about keeping my intake of fat and cholesterol down." So, in order to give this concept some grounding, and "tone" any sagging credibility, I need to dispel some of the prevailing mythology around food. In the next chapter, I'll do just that.

11

Just the Facts, Ma'am

I would imagine that by this point in your life you have determined the identity of the Tooth Fairy. We pass through many stages of development in this wonderful adventure we call life, but some of the myths we live with are much more difficult to change than others. Identifying and challenging these myths, however, is vital, because only the truth will set us free. There are myths galore that have grown up around health and nutrition. In this chapter, we'll confront just a few of the more common and potentially dangerous ones. So, let's mount up—it's time to slay a few dragons!

Myth #1: Eating fat makes you fat.

To understand why this massive myth about the fat that we eat came about, we first of all need to take a look at the caloric value of fat. One calorie is defined as the amount of energy needed to increase the temperature of one gram of water by one degree Celsius. Thus, the calorie is a measure of energy. Since the body needs energy to function, nutrition scientists wanted to determine how much energy is available from each of the three food groups: carbohydrates, proteins and fats. So, they took various representative foods from each food group and placed them in what's known as a Bomb Calorimeter: a device that is able to measure how much energy is released when the chemical bonds in food are broken down. They found that proteins and carbohydrates have four calories per gram, and fat has nine calories per gram (Rinzler, 1999).

Soon after these measurements were made, we found ourselves in trouble as a calorie-counting society. A little knowledge can truly be dangerous sometimes. You see, from these measurements, we concluded that fat is almost twice as calorie intense as proteins or carbohydrates. So, we decided it was better to avoid fat—thinking that if we don't burn it, then we'll store all those extra calories. Yes, we do store extra fat; and, yes, energy that is stored or burned can be thought of in terms of calories. But fat is also used as a *building block* to manufacture cell walls, hormones, antioxidants, and other important molecules. It is erroneous to think of building blocks in terms of calories. Therefore, it is also erroneous to say that fat is "calorie intensive" to the body, since not all of the potential calories are used or stored for energy.

For example, if you eat a sandwich worth 300 calories, that means it's possible to get 300 calories of energy from that sandwich in a test tube. In the body, however, not all of those 300 calories can be used for energy because not all protein and fat gets burned up for energy. Most of the protein will be broken down into amino acids and then rebuilt into the protein molecules we need in the body. Some of the fat will be used to make hormones, vitamin D and cell membranes, among other things. The carbohydrates in that sandwich will supply us with quick energy, but can also be stored for future energy needs in the form of glycogen (a good thing) or body fat (not such a good thing).

What does all this mean? Well, it means for one thing that you should stop counting calories, because the caloric value of fat is not what it seems. I would like to be able to tell you exactly how many calories from fat you use as building blocks and how many you use for energy. Unfortunately, the research hasn't been done and no one knows. Also, these percentages would likely vary according to such factors as a person's age, activity level and weight. All I *can* tell you is that we are neither test tubes nor Bomb Calorimeters. We are human beings, and besides burning food for energy, we also use food to rebuild tissue. We cannot simply judge fat from a caloric perspective. We need to replenish the body with the fat it needs to maintain cellular function. While eating an excessive number of calories will always remain a bad idea, most of our emphasis should be placed on choosing quality (some kinds of fat are good for us, others extremely bad) instead of merely reducing quantity. But whether we eat beneficial fats or harmful fats, the fat we eat does not equal the fat we wear on our bodies.

If you still absolutely insist on counting the number of fat calories you consume, then consider quality as well as quantity. Later in this chapter you'll learn about quality. As far as quantity goes, the good fats should make up about 30% of your caloric intake. Volume-wise, this looks to be about 1–2 tablespoons of total fat per meal. For instance, if you eat 1,800 calories in a day, some 540 calories (4 1/2 tablespoons) should come from fat. We'll talk more about that in the next chapter.

To give you another sneak preview of what's coming up: when you eat from the Longevity Pyramid, which serves as a graphic summary at the end of this chapter, you should never have to count calories at all—whether they're from fats, proteins or carbohydrates. Why? Well, are you ever in danger of eating too much salad? Have you ever watched someone eat a sack full of apples or a whole head of broccoli? How many hard-boiled eggs could you eat at one sitting? Maybe you could eat two or three, but certainly not ten, because you'd get sick to your stomach. Now ask yourself if you could finish a bar of chocolate or a bag of chips at one sitting? How big a bowl of pasta would be enough to comfort you on a cold winter day? Calorie counting is necessary only when you eat processed foods. The body has a feedback mechanism in place, designed to keep it from overeating, but this protection only works with Mother Nature's foods or, that is to say, with what our Stone Age ancestors ate. This mechanism has not adapted to man-made or processed foods, so it's no wonder that we tend to overeat. Cave dwellers never ate chocolate, chips or pasta. So, if you can't theoretically "hunt it, fish it, pick it or milk it," then you'd better worry about counting it.

Myth #2: Eating cholesterol should be kept to a minimum.[1]

Physicians, health organizations, food packaging, health articles and books—almost everywhere you turn, the recommendation is still to reduce the amount of cholesterol we

---

[1] To truly appreciate this myth, I would recommend that you read Dr. Schwarzbein's account of working with patients on increasing their intake of dietary fat and reducing processed carbohydrates, in her book *The Schwarzbein Principle* (available online at www.hci-online.com).

get in our diet. Dietary cholesterol is a special kind of fat found only in animal fat such as meat, poultry, shellfish and dairy, and as you'll soon find out, it's a necessary component of every cell in the body. But *dietary* cholesterol is not the same as *serum* cholesterol, and herein lies the origin of the myth. Furthermore, just as many people with total serum cholesterol levels below 200 die of heart attacks as those with total serum cholesterol levels above 200 (Schwarzbein and Deville, 1999). So the myth is based on *two false assumptions*:

1. Total serum cholesterol is always a good indicator of heart disease.
2. Serum cholesterol is somehow related to dietary cholesterol.

How did our society become so obsessed with measuring serum cholesterol levels and avoiding dietary cholesterol? For at least part of the answer, let's look to a number of studies done in the late 1970s and early 1980s that were designed on the flawed premise that the fat and cholesterol that an individual eats determine his or her serum cholesterol level. Working from this key assumption, scientists set out to investigate whether serum cholesterol was a determining risk factor for heart disease.

One such study, which was published in the journal *Lancet* back in 1981, has made a lasting impression on the medical community. The researchers studied 1,232 men in Oslo, Norway for five years to determine the effect of diet and smoking on heart disease (Hjermann et al., 1981). The men were split into two groups—a control group and an intervention group. The members of the control group were left to their own devices, whereas the intervention group participants were given lots of advice around diet and smoking. Now, some of the advice that was given at that time would seem dated to us today. For instance, participants were told to eat margarine as a way of reducing cholesterol in their diet. Today, we know that margarine is full of harmful trans fats. We'll talk more about harmful fats later in this chapter, but my point here is that as I evaluated this and other studies, I repeatedly encountered the words "improved diet," even though the researchers hadn't actually established what constitutes such an "improved diet." A second point of contention with this particular study is that the researchers asked the intervention group to change five variables. They were asked to:

- reduce cholesterol and saturated fat intake
- reduce sugar intake
- increase poly-unsaturated fat intake
- decrease smoking
- decrease alcohol consumption

The reason this study is considered so significant is that the members of the intervention group reduced their overall risk of heart disease by 47%. But the real clincher is that the individuals of this group had cut back on their tobacco consumption by 45%. The researchers did a lot of statistical analysis, trying to dissect which of the above five factors had the greatest influence on heart disease. They did some fancy math and found that serum cholesterol levels were a stronger indicator of heart disease than smoking. *But they hadn't asked the participants to change their serum choles-*

terol. So this begs the question: how or why did serum cholesterol change? And here comes the leap of faith. In response to this study, the scientific community at large *assumed* that serum cholesterol could be determined by the intake of fat and cholesterol in the diet, even though there was no real evidence to support that notion in the study. In fact, we now know that smoking can increase insulin levels, which in turn can increase serum cholesterol.

Had that study been done today, we would immediately see that it was those darn cigarettes; we now know that every time a person smokes, it increases the risk of heart disease (Cook et al., 1986). Nonetheless, this dated study, which had been designed to change *five* possible variables, was interpreted to mean that dietary fat and cholesterol are the *only* variables that increase the risk of heart disease. Sadly, it's taking decades to reverse this myth.

I, for one, am ready to look at some facts about cholesterol. Here is something we are absolutely sure of—cholesterol is a necessary component of every cell in the body.

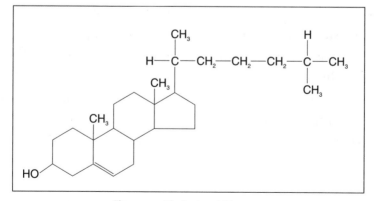

Figure 15. Cholesterol Diagram

Cholesterol is a single molecule, as shown in *Figure 15*. However, medical professionals and researchers throw the word "cholesterol" around, when it can refer to many different entities.

For instance, the work of many scientists, including Nobel Laureates Brown and Goldstein, has revealed that *serum* cholesterol—cholesterol in the blood—refers to a whole host of far more complicated macromolecules called "lipoproteins." Lipoproteins contain hundreds of those relatively simple cholesterol molecules we looked at in the diagram, as well as hundreds of fat molecules and large protein molecules. Unfortunately, calling it "serum cholesterol" has set us up to think that there should be a direct correlation between cholesterol that is consumed—dietary cholesterol—and cholesterol that is found in the blood—serum cholesterol. The term could also suggest that serum cholesterol is one type of molecule, when in fact it represents many molecules. Serum *cholesterol* would more appropriately be called serum *lipoproteins*.

You've probably been told about your HDLs, LDLs (see *Figure 16* on facing page) and VLDLs, and that your serum cholesterol is the sum of these things. Well, it is actually much more complicated[2], but suffice it to say that each of these lipoproteins has an origin and a purpose that is different from its brothers and sisters. There are many factors that influence the levels at which they are found in the blood. For instance, it is the job of HDLs to pick up cholesterol released into the plasma from dying cells.

---

[2] Serum cholesterol is the sum of many plasma lipoproteins including chylomicrons, chylomicron remnants, very-low-density lipoproteins (VLDL), intermediate-density lipoproteins (IDL), low-density lipoproteins (LDL) and high-density lipoproteins (HDL). While some of these are formed from dietary fats and cholesterol, there are other factors that affect total serum cholesterol (Stryer, 1988).

You might have heard that your LDLs should be low; but LDL is not the culprit—it's gotten a bum rap! It's the LDLs that have been oxidized by free radicals that you need to worry about. We know that a diet rich in vitamin E can protect LDL, and that this fat-soluble vitamin is a component of LDL. Indeed, when vitamin E-rich, whole food is consumed, the risk of heart disease declines (Kushi et al., 1996). Because of the subtleties inherent in understanding the various components of serum cholesterol, experts in the field have yet to agree whether any or all of them are good indicators of any disease (Hayashi and Nakamura, 1991; Kannel and Gordon, 1982). We know that at very high or very low levels, these molecules are saying, "Hey, something is wrong here." But by then, you probably don't need a doctor to tell you that you are sick. Serum cholesterol is also a very late indicator of disease. For example, my father suffered with heart disease and his total serum cholesterol was never over 200. However, he had been a smoker. He is far from being an isolated example. In fact, just as many people suffer from heart disease who have a total serum

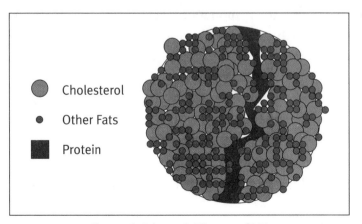

Figure 16. Schematic Diagram of LDL

cholesterol count of less than 200 as do those with a count greater than 200.

Elevated serum cholesterol is usually a problem related more to diet (one that is poor in antioxidants and rich in sugar) and lifestyle (smoking, lack of exercise) than it is to bad cholesterol-processing genes. A very small percentage of people do actually have a genetic disorder called "familial hypercholesterolemia," which is a serious condition where they lack the receptor for processing LDL, and requires medication; but this genetic defect is certainly not the norm.

Many people who've been told that they have high serum cholesterol are running around avoiding dietary cholesterol. This is because they are convinced that they have bad genes, when what they most likely have are bad habits around diet and lifestyle. And I don't doubt that many of us *have* inherited bad habits. Drastically reducing dietary cholesterol does not lower health risks. The focus should be on eating more vegetables, eating healthy fats and limiting processed sugars, quitting smoking and adding a regular program of moderate exercise. These are the key ways in which to build a healthy body and thereby reduce serum cholesterol.

Eat an abundance of Mother Nature's whole foods–even those that naturally come with some cholesterol. You can trust your liver to figure out what it is that your body needs. The liver is the great clearinghouse of the body. Nobel Prize winner Pablo Neruda has written in his *Ode to the Liver*:

There, inside, you filter and apportion
you separate and divide,
you multiply and lubricate
you raise and gather
he threads and the grams of life...

The liver is certainly interested in the amount of dietary cholesterol you take in at each meal, because cholesterol plays an essential role in your body's health. For example, cholesterol:

- is needed for the integrity of all your cell membranes
- insulates your nerve cells
- is a building block for vitamin D, made when sunlight hits the fat just under your skin
- enables your gall bladder to make bile acids—digestive chemicals that allow you to absorb fat-soluble nutrients such as vitamin A, vitamin D, vitamin E and vitamin K
- is used as a building block for making important hormones such as estrogen and testosterone

You can see why the liver likes to keep tabs on dietary cholesterol. After the liver receives a small sample of your meal through the portal vein, it will take note of how much cholesterol is in your blood. If there is little or no cholesterol then the liver takes it upon itself to *make* cholesterol. Again, this is one of those fundamental concepts that "popular medicine" has stepped over. I'll explain what I mean by that.

The enzymatic reaction that commits the body to the synthesis of cholesterol—called the "committed step"—is catalyzed by the enzyme 3-hydroxy-3-methylglutaryl CoA reductase (HMG CoA reductase). The bad news is that, once HMG CoA reductase gets going, it won't stop unless we get enough cholesterol. For all it knows, the body is in the middle of a cholesterol famine, and it will do all that it can to deal with that crisis. If we were to continue to restrict our intake of cholesterol, the production of cholesterol, meal after meal, could cause serum cholesterol to rise. Conversely, eating cholesterol inhibits this enzyme. So, when we include cholesterol in our diet, the liver will produce less of it.

Now, drug companies know all of this biochemistry. That's why they market expensive "statin" drugs that inhibit the action of HMG CoA reductase. But the funny thing is that HMG CoA reductase would not be active in the first place if we had eaten dietary cholesterol. Statin drugs rank as one of the Top Ten prescription drugs, and by 1999, had already generated $9.2 billion in sales (Wollschlaeger, 2001). Many of the potential side effects of these statin drugs are being discussed in the scientific literature and some have even made headline news; but such discussion and disclosure is not the norm. The information that physicians receive on the potential and/or actual side effects of drugs is not usually so up-to-date.

In a double-blind, placebo-controlled study[3], published back in 1993, statin drugs were shown to dramatically reduce (by 50–54%) levels of the very important antioxidant, Coenzyme Q10 (CoQ10). Like cholesterol, CoQ10 is also manufactured in the liver and shares the same "committed step" reaction catalyzed by HMG-CoA reductase as

---

[3] Double-blind, placebo-controlled studies refer to studies where neither the investigator nor the subject actually knows who is getting the placebo and who is getting the item being tested.

the synthesis of cholesterol. *Thus, when statin drugs inhibit HMG-CoA reductase in an effort to reduce serum cholesterol, they also cause a reduction in CoQ10.* CoQ10 is one of the antioxidants that we can make in the body. Among other things, *CoQ10 is essential to the proper function of the mitochondria[4], which are, in turn, responsible for the production of energy within each and every one of our cells.*

So, here is a drug that we think is very specific in its action—that is, it inhibits just one enzyme in the body. Yet, it can also affect the lifespan of the body at a cellular level by reducing blood levels of CoQ10. In other words, statin drugs may drain the batteries of all of the cells in the body, especially those of muscle tissue, which is particularly rich in mitochondria.

The breakdown of muscle mitochondria, in fact, may be at the heart of a recent news article suggesting the possible need to put a warning label on statin drugs. The article said, "A rare but deadly side effect of the popular cholesterol-lowering drugs known as statins has killed and injured more people than the government has acknowledged." The side effect they are referring to is muscle breakdown, known as rhabdomyolysis[5]. "Doctors and patients are grossly unin-

---

[4] CoQ10 is the naturally-occurring form of ubiquinone in humans. Ubiquinone is essential to mitochondrial function.

[5] My friend Dr. David Bove and I hypothesize that as a result of CoQ10 being inhibited by statin drugs, the electron transport chain and oxidative phosphorylation in the mitochondria would become impaired, depleting ATP production. This depletion of ATP would lead to changes in membrane potential resulting in increased intracellular Na+ and a resultant increase in intracellular Ca++. Such changes promote the activity of intracellular proteolytic enzymes that cause cellular destruction and consequent muscle breakdown. It actually becomes a feed forward cycle as the increased intracellular Na+ activates the Na+/K+ ATPase pump, utilizing significant amounts of ATP and further depleting its stores, leading to further breakdown. This hypothesis is partly inspired by Dr. David Perlmutter's construct related to neurodegenerative disease. He talks of the feed forward cycle of glutamate stimulation of the NMDA receptor leading to Ca++ influx and mitochondrial degeneration, which feeds on itself as the diminished ATP changes the membrane potential, making it more susceptible to glutamate stimulation.

formed about this," says Sidney Wolfe, director of Public Citizen's Health Research Group (Sternberg, 2001).

Now, the physicians who *are* aware of this possible effect often recommend taking a CoQ10 supplement in conjunction with statin drugs. While I advocate taking certain supplements to make up for general nutrient deficiencies, I do not advocate trying to use supplements as a way of offsetting any harm that may be done by pharmaceuticals. This can lead to a false sense of security about the use of certain drugs. Even if this strategy of simultaneously taking CoQ10 in supplement form to maintain CoQ10 levels while taking statin drugs were to work, there would be other side effects to consider.

Some studies have found that those who take statin drugs to lower their cholesterol seem more likely to die from tragic causes, such as car accidents and suicides. Such data would indicate that these drugs may cause a loss of mental acuity (Haney, 1997). Another line of investigation has shown that statin drugs can suppress the immune system (Kwak et al., 2000). The authors of the immune system study actually seemed to be excited by this finding, since statin drugs may have an application for patients with organ transplants. In order to accept a foreign organ, transplant recipients need to suppress their own immune systems. The authors think statin drugs could be particularly well suited for this purpose. But what of the 4+ million Americans who take statin drugs and *aren't* getting an organ transplant? Do they also benefit from having their immune systems suppressed? In any case, all of these side effects could simply be avoided by refusing to rely on these drugs in the first place. As I suggested earlier, we could trust the liver to regulate cholesterol levels, and eat dietary cholesterol. Enough of those re-constituted pseudo-eggs in a carton! Go ahead and crack some organic eggs! Eat them every day, if you want! And you'll cook them in a small amount of butter, too, if you know what's good for you! Sound too good to be true? Stay tuned, if you want even more justification.

From where I stand, much of the current momentum in the sale of statin drugs can be attributed to a ball that started rolling several decades ago, back in the late 1970s and early 1980s. It was then that the faulty assumption was made that serum cholesterol is the direct result of eating dietary cholesterol and fats. This is a perfect example of how the vicious cycle of the Default Health Program can perpetuate the use of pharmaceuticals. Years of unnecessary and arguably dangerous drug use could have been avoided by revisiting the fundamental concepts of biochemistry. That is, long before this whole "anti-fat, anti-cholesterol movement" in medicine got started, we'd already determined that the liver would make cholesterol if it were missing from the diet. Sadly, the original research against dietary cholesterol not only lacked good evidence, but also wasn't even grounded in previously known facts.

A healthy alternative for people worried about cholesterol may be eating more vegetables and fruits, as well as supplementation with Juice Plus+®. For instance, we talked about how oxidative damage can turn normal LDLs into damaged LDLs in the serum. Phytonutrients such as resveratrols, flavonoids and polyphenols can protect LDL molecules from oxidative damage (Fremont et al., 1999).

Oxidized LDLs compromise the health of the endothelium, which is the thin layer of tissue that lines all of our arteries and veins.

Investigators in the field of cardiovascular disease believe that the health of the endothelial tissue is paramount for protection against stroke and heart disease. And we have quite a bit of endothelial tissue to protect. If I were to take all of your endothelial tissue and spread it out, it would cover about six tennis courts.

Two leading researchers in this field, Dr. Gary Plotnick and Dr. Robert Vogel, have developed an interesting way to test the health of the endothelial tissue. They give their subjects a typical McDonald's® breakfast—in order to see how they fare afterwards. Guess what? For at least six hours afterwards, arteries are unable to expand properly in order to handle the blood flow needed during physical or emotional stress. These researchers believe that this resulting constriction may be one reason why people who already have "clogged" arteries so often suffer heart attacks soon after eating a meal high in damaged fats. They reason that the oxidative stress created by eating such a meal is what causes the constriction. Indeed, Drs. Plotnick and Vogel suggest that taking high doses of antioxidants such as vitamin C and vitamin E can prevent this type of constriction (Plotnick et al., 1997).

However, for the reasons that I discussed in *Chapter Nine*, I wouldn't recommend a daily, high dose of any antioxidant. You may get some specific benefits, but there are other costs associated with isolated, fragmented supplements. Fortunately, these same researchers have found that the whole food based Juice Plus+® products give the same kinds of results in protecting the endothelium (Plotnick et al., 2001). Taking Juice Plus+® provides significant protection for the endothelium as it deals with that meal from McDonald's®. Now I'm not recommending that you throw caution to the wind, and then just pop some Juice Plus+®; but this test does show that proper antioxidant protection can do a lot to prevent the damage of oxidative stress. And besides, whether you eat at McDonald's® or not, you still need to protect yourself from the oxidative stress that is constantly coming at you from so many directions. Remember the antioxidant balancing act in *Figure 8, Chapter Eight*? If we want to guard our health, we must constantly be involved in an intricate balancing act between free radicals and antioxidants. And it appears that as far as your circulatory system is concerned, Juice Plus+® offers additional support against oxidative stress.

Thus, the combination of appropriate amounts of dietary cholesterol with these whole food based supplements offers a much safer option for proper cholesterol regulation, such that:

- You provide your body with the cholesterol it needs.
- You then protect that cholesterol, using powerful phytonutrients.

It seems to me that given all of the knowledge, food choices and supplements available to us today, no one should have to suffer from the consequences of high levels of oxidized LDLs in the blood. Nor should it be necessary for millions of people to be taking statin drugs to lower their cholesterol. It's easy to forget sometimes, but the body is actually designed to process cholesterol, provided it's given the raw materials it needs to work with.

Myth #3: You should cook with unsaturated fats and avoid eating saturated fats.

To expose this myth, we'll first need to have at least a basic understanding of the three kinds of fats found in nature: saturated, mono-unsaturated and poly-unsaturated. While the word "fat" is generally used to describe a wide variety of molecules, these three adjectives specifically describe the three kinds of "fatty acids" that are pertinent to our discussion of fats in food. These fatty acids are made up of carbon and hydrogen atoms. Carbon atoms have the potential to make four bonds. Within this "hydrocarbon chain," not all the carbon atoms use up all four bonds to bind to four other molecules. It is within this bonding

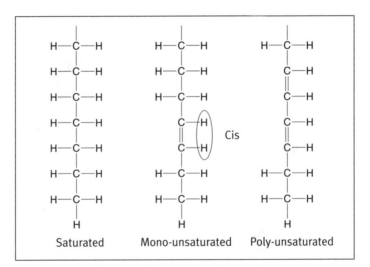

Figure 17. Three types of fatty acids

process that the differentiation occurs among the three types of fatty acids. Sometimes there are double bonds between carbon atoms. When there are no double bonds, it means the hydrocarbon chain is "saturated" with hydrogen atoms. If there is one double bond, then the chain is said to be "mono-unsaturated," because it has the potential to break the double bond and thereby allow each of the two carbons that were participating in the double bond to take on an additional hydrogen atom. If there are two or more double bonds, then we have a "poly-unsaturated" chain.

The thing about these double bonds is that in nature they occur in what is called a "cis" configuration. Cis means "same-side." So, while the preceding diagram (*Figure 17*) shows a stick figure version of the chain, the more descriptive *Figure 18* (below) shows how these cis bonds create kinks in the chain. Notice that the kinks always bend to the same side. These kinky poly-unsaturated fatty acids provide a very

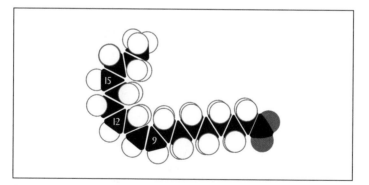

Figure 18. Space-filling model of linoliate, a poly-unsaturated fatty acid with three cis double bonds; the carbon atoms are in black, hydrogen in white and oxygen in grey. There are cis double bonds between carbons 9 and 10, between 12 and 13, and between 15 and 16.
Reprinted with permission of W.H. Freeman and Company from BIOCHEMISTRY by Lubert Stryer. ©1988 by Lubert Stryer.

useful purpose for the membrane of every cell in the body.

The cell membrane and the membranes of all the various compartments inside the cells, called organelles, are made up of what are called phospholipids. These are large molecules that have one head and two of these hydrocarbon chains that form the tails. The head of a phospholipid molecule likes water, while the tails repel water. Wanting to repel the aqueous solution inside and outside each cell, the phospholipid tails arrange themselves in two layers that face each other to make the membrane of a cell as shown in *Figure 19.*

Imbedded within cell membranes are various kinds of enzymes. Enzymes are proteins that catalyze chemical reactions in the body, such as "receptor" proteins that detect incoming messages and "channel" proteins that are specialized passageways for particular chemicals. The proper functioning of these enzymes requires a fluid membrane so that

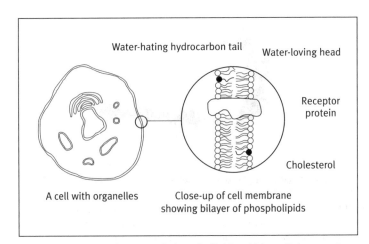

Figure 19. Schematic diagram of phospholipids within cellular membranes

the enzymes are free to move and function, and do not get stuck in one position, which would make them useless. That is where the cis double bond kinks become so important. If there were no kinks, the membranes would be made up of phospholipids with very straight tails. This would make for a more compact or rigid membrane. A rigid membrane is a sick membrane, because the enzymes are not free to move and function properly. So, there you have it: the basic rationale for the inclusion of poly-unsaturated fats in our diet.

The Yin and Yang[6] of poly-unsaturated fats is that while they are critical to our health and vitality, they are also fragile molecules that need protection, or else they may become damaged, and thereby harmful to us. This potentially dangerous transformation takes place when the hydrocarbon tails are exposed to heat and free radicals. Heat creates "hydrogenated" and "trans" fats. Free radicals make rancid fats called "lipid peroxides" (lipid means fat). I'll explain each of these so that you can better understand why and how to avoid eating these damaged fats. Much of the past confusion around fat—whether it's good for you or not—has to do with not fully appreciating the fragile nature of good poly-unsaturated fats. As we learn more, a complete picture is emerging.

Poly + HEAT = Hydrogenated Fats & TRANS Fats

Heating unsaturated fats can add hydrogen atoms to the

---

[6] In Chinese philosophy, Yin and Yang represent all the opposite principles one finds in the universe. For instance, under Yang are the principles such as maleness, the sun, creation, heat, light, and so on, and under Yin are the principles of femaleness, the moon, completion, cold, darkness, and so on. I think of poly-unsaturated fats as dynamic molecules that allow us to harness energy, make incredibly complex cellular structures and provide molecules for cellular communication. Yet, when they are unprotected from heat, light and oxygen, they can quench life and cause cellular chaos.

double bonds and these *hydrogenated* tails will have fewer kinks in them. Hydrogenated fats are similar to saturated fats in that their respective tails are saturated with hydrogen atoms. Now, I don't go out of my way to avoid whole foods that naturally contain some saturated fat. I assume that there must be a good reason for the saturated fat in whole food, even though scientists haven't figured out what it is yet[7]. On the other hand, I see no reason to eat man-made solid fats. Why eat hydrogenated fat when I could be eating the original, unprocessed, kinky, poly-unsaturated fats that could serve as important structural fat for my body? In other words, why insult my body with man-made, toxic crackers or bread, when I could be eating a salad with good fat in the dressing instead? Add to this the fact that there is an inherent danger in this man-made process. Some of the fats become trans fats instead of hydrogenated fats.

The introduction of heat during processing can flip the cis double bond around into a *trans* configuration, where

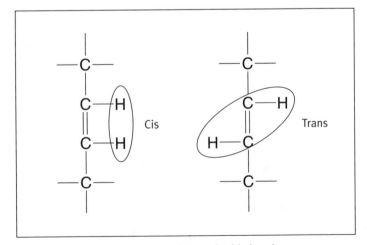

Figure 20. Cis and trans double bonds

_____
[7] For instance, it would be interesting to study what blend of saturated and unsaturated fats makes for a healthy cell membrane that is not too fluid or too solid—and how we would best achieve this optimum ratio through diet.

the kink is now in a direction that does not occur in natural fats. Since trans fats don't occur in natural foods, we don't have enzymes to break down or process or utilize trans fats, and so the body becomes littered with these sticky fats. That's what makes trans fats the worst kind of fats that you can eat. That said, if you still want to increase your intake of these trans fats in order to litter your insides with grease spots, go ahead and chow down on margarine, vegetable shortening, doughnuts, crackers, cookies, chips, cakes, pies, breads and fried foods. The downside to this diet regimen will be the deposit of solid fats in your arteries, liver and other organs. In other words, don't think that those unprocessed trans fats will be eliminated from your body and that you can just flush your sins down the toilet! Trans fats will stick to your insides and eventually cause heart attacks, stroke and circulatory occlusions. A double whammy is that these foods are also poor choices as far as micronutrient content. Dr. Walter C. Willett, the nutritionist from Harvard whom I mentioned earlier, calls trans fats the "biggest food-processing disaster in U.S. history" and blames trans fats for at least 30,000 premature deaths per year (Carper, 2001).

When corn oil is heated to make margarine, the poly-unsaturated fats in the oil either become hydrogenated or, worse, they become trans fats. So even though you may have started out with a helpful poly-unsaturated fat, the processing makes that fat harmful. According to the Framingham Heart Study, each teaspoon of margarine consumed in a day can boost a man's chance of coronary heart disease by 10%. In other words, 3 teaspoons a day would increase risk by 30%. Eating the same amount of butter does not appear to increase risk of coronary heart disease (Gillman et al., 1997). The moral of that story is that butter, with all its cholesterol and saturated fats, is still better.

You may be equally confused by all of the recommen-dations about which kind of oil to cook in. *In general, cooking with any kind of fat is not a good idea.* But if you do cook with fat, remember that saturated fats are the only ones which contain no double bonds; so, there is minimal potential to damage them through heat. A second-best choice is mono-unsaturated fats, with only one double bond that could potentially get damaged by heat. Here is a list of fats that are acceptable for cooking under low heat:

Butter	Sour Cream
Coconut Oil	Avocado Oil
Olive Oil	Rice Oil
Canola Oil	Hazelnut Oil
Grapeseed Oil	Oat Oil
Mustard Oil	Peanut Oil
Nutmeg Oil	Poultry Fat
Cocoa Butter	

On the other hand, unsaturated fats, with their double bonds have the potential to become trans fats. So, cook with a small amount of butter or coconut oil and use low heat. Then, if you want to, drizzle your good (unheated) unsaturated fats on top afterwards. Salads are another food on which you can drizzle your unsaturated fats.

Even when you're dedicated to making healthy choices, it's important to stay alert and read labels. Does the label on your favorite salad dressing say the words "partially hydrogenated oil"? If it does, you could be turning an otherwise healthy salad into a toxic lunch. Here are some good fats to use cold in salad dressings, in smoothies or taken as supplements. Make sure when you buy them that they were cold processed and were also *stored* cold, in dark containers, prior to purchase:

Flaxseed Oil	Salmon Oil
Borage Oil	Sardine Oil
Wheat Germ Oil	Herring Oil
Primrose Oil	

And remember to store these fats in dark bottles and in cold places at home as well, opened or not. In time, the vegetable oils in clear bottles sitting at the store and then in your home will go bad. This also applies to salad dressings that are stored at room temperature. It's the Yin and Yang of poly-unsaturated fats. For cooking, avoid using the following unsaturated vegetable oils:

Corn Oil	Sesame Oil
Safflower Oil	Walnut Oil
Sunflower Oil	Poppyseed oil
Cottonseed Oil	Soybean Oil

These fats are generally bad because excessive heat is used to extract the oil from the plants. Sometimes cold-pressed alternatives may be found, but then the omega-3 to omega-6 fats are usually out of balance, as you'll soon learn, so why bother?

Myth #4: We should eat a low-fat diet.

Fat is greatly misunderstood. I am repeatedly frustrated when I travel and all I can find is low-fat milk and yogurt in airports, convenience stores and strip malls. When was the last time you had luxurious, creamy, whole yogurt? Who needs the slimy, processed fruit (excess sugar) when you can have the fat! Our birthright to eat dietary fat is being replaced with sugar, which you'll soon learn is not such a great substitute, and our hips are showing the result. A low-fat diet is especially a problem for children. If I'm not careful to make sure that my children get their fat and avoid sugar at all costs, I can see a difference in their behavior within twenty-four hours. I have seen children suffering from a multitude of skin diseases and being given myriad pharmaceuticals in an attempt to combat the problem. It is not uncommon for skin problems to appear after a child is weaned from fat-rich breast milk. The first remedy to try is goat milk and, perhaps, an essential fatty acid supplement geared for kids. Typically, young children are getting too many carbohydrates in juices, pastas, cereals, breads, crackers and the like, and not getting enough protein or fat. Adding a tablespoon of flaxseed oil or borage oil to any solid foods in their diet is also an easy way to handle this lack of dietary fat. Within a few weeks of adding these fats back to their diet, parents should see a noticeable improvement in the condition of the problem skin. In any case, I would first try to rule out nutritional deficiencies before subjecting children to strong pharmaceuticals.

Here are the common warning signs that your diet may be deficient in dietary fat (Schwarzbein and Deville, 1999):

Addictive behavior	Insomnia
Brittle nails	Loss of lean mass
Constipation	Mood disorders
Dry, limp, thinning hair	Scaly, itchy skin
Excess body fat	Sugar cravings
Infertility	

It is apparent from the list that when there is not enough fat in the diet, one of the key building blocks for the body is missing. For instance, poly-unsaturated fatty acids are important building blocks for a multitude of important chemicals in the body, such as hormones and antioxidants. The body makes poly-unsaturated fatty acids from four kinds of fatty acid precursors (building blocks):

- palmitoleate (is the precursor for omega-7 fatty acids)
- oleate (omega-9 precursor)
- linoleate (omega-6 precursor)
- linolenate (omega-3 precursor)

The omega-number is just a fancy designation, referring to how far away the first, cis-double bond is from the very end of the fatty acid tail. Of these, the last two, linoleate (LA) and linolenate (LNA), cannot be synthesized in the body; and they are considered *essential* fatty acids. So, if we try to eliminate fats altogether in our diet, we will not consume enough of these essential fatty acids for our bodies to function properly. Without sufficient intake of poly-unsaturated fats, the saturated fats will take their place in the membranes. This makes for membranes that are less fluid, and, therefore, less healthy. When the receptors and other proteins get stuck in a rigid membrane, the cell loses the ability to communicate with the rest of the body. Furthermore, the body cannot manufacture the hormones and other chemicals it needs to function. Thus, a diet lacking in essential fats necessarily leads to an increase in body fat, premature aging, and disease.

It is very important for pregnant and lactating women to get the essential fats they need, while avoiding the damaged fats. Edema and high blood pressure are complications that arise from eating a diet rich in trans fats during pregnancy. These same trans fats can also pass in the mother's blood through the placenta to the developing fetus, having a harmful effect on fetal programming. Even after birth, a nursing mother can pass trans fats on to her baby in her breast milk, which can diminish the infant's visual acuity and brain development (Hornstra, 2000). Meanwhile, poly-unsaturated fats in the placenta and breast milk are incorporated into the baby's brain at a fast and furious pace. While a developing brain likes to see poly-unsaturated fatty acids with lots of kinks, it doesn't want to be littered with trans fats.

To further complicate matters, not only do we need LA and LNA in our diet, we also need these essential fatty acids in the correct ratios. Two important changes occurred at the turn of the last century that altered the types and ratios of fats we started to consume in our diet. First, the invention of the Expeller press technology marked the beginning of the vegetable-oil industry (Kirschenbauer, 1960). With time, vegetable oil extraction from seed grew more efficient and economical. By the 1940s, food manufacturers started to use these oils in pre-packaged foods in order to increase their shelf life. Such processing introduced harmful hydrogenated and trans fats into our diets for the first time.

The second important change was the shift in modern agriculture toward feeding grain to domestic livestock, instead of allowing them to graze freely on grass and the bugs on the grass. Feed grains are rich in the omega-6 precursor LA, but low in the omega-3 precursor LNA. Further down the food chain, foods that come from animals fed a grain-based diet, such as meat, dairy and eggs are also rich in LA-derived omega-6 fatty acids, but are missing many of the equally desirable omega-3 fatty acids derived from LNA.

Thus, most of our food has also lost the balance between the two types of essential fatty acids. The business of modern agriculture emphasizes quantity over quality. This bottom line has pulled the Western diet away from the balance of omega-3 to omega-6 fatty acids in vegetables, animal meats, eggs and fish. For instance, when you buy beef in the store, it has small or undetectable amounts of LNA, which is the important precursor for omega-3 fatty acids. If you were to hunt down a deer for dinner, that wild meat would have much more LNA than its domestic counterpart. Domesticated cattle are fed grains rich in omega-6 fatty acids in order to achieve maximum size in the least amount of time. The result is that domestic beef has almost undetectable amounts of omega-3 fatty acids. By contrast, deer that can forage freely on wild fern and moss produce meat that contains many more omega-3 fatty acids (Crawford et al., 1969). If you can track down a source of grass-fed beef in your town, I suggest the benefits outweigh any inconvenience. Similarly, yolks from the eggs of free-

roaming chickens have a ratio of omega-6 to omega-3 of
4 to 3. Compare that to U.S. Department of Agriculture
standard grain-fed eggs with a ratio of 194 to 10
(Simopoulos and Salem, 1992).

A balance closer to 1 omega-6 to 1 omega-3 existed in
our diet during our long genetic history of millions of years.
In only about 100 years, since the invention of vegetable-oil
expression machines and the trend toward grain-fed livestock, there has been an unprecedented shift in the balance
of essential fats in the American diet. To my knowledge,
there is no precedent for such a drastic change in diet over
such a short period of time.

So, is there any evidence that we need to re-establish
this balance of omega-3 and omega-6? It seems so.
Experimental studies confirm that the proper combination of
the two fats, omega-3 and omega-6, has the maximal effect
on lowering blood pressure, improving the serum lipid profile and reducing atherosclerosis in animal studies
(Kochetova et al., 1993). As I've mentioned, heart disease is
the biggest killer in America, as well as in many other industrialized countries with diets typically lacking in omega-3
fatty acids. Meanwhile, low rates of heart disease are found
in Greenland Eskimos and the Japanese, who eat a diet rich
in fish oil with a high content of omega-3 fats (Das, 2000).
A diet that contains wild fish has a more balanced omega-3
to omega-6 essential fatty acid ratio; in contrast, farm fish
that are fed the products of modern agriculture have more
omega-6 fats. Over the last thirty years, evidence has been
mounting that omega-3 fatty acids are good for the heart.
The American Heart Association (AHA) is convinced

enough to recommend eating two 3-ounce servings of fish a week.

What if you don't care for fish or it is difficult to find a fresh supply. Is fish oil supplementation a viable option? So far, the question of fish oil supplementation has been a little tricky—it may be too easy to get too much of a good thing with a supplement. One of the benefits of omega-3 fatty acids is that they lower the risk of blood clots, which can trigger a heart attack; but the AHA is worried that too much omega-3 may cause internal bleeding. Yet, it has been shown that 3 grams of omega-3 fatty acids a day, taken in supplement form, afford the benefits without the risk of an increase in bleeding time (Blonk et al., 1990).

A convincing case was made for supplementation by a group of British researchers who studied 11,324 heart attack patients for two years. The patients were divided into random groups. The first group received vitamin E; the second also received vitamin E, as well as fish oil; the third group received fish oil only; and the fourth received a placebo. After the two-year period, only the two groups that had received fish oil supplements showed a significant 17% reduction in their risk of a second heart attack (Fish oil study, 1999).

What are the potential side effects of fish oil capsules? According to the American Heart Association, they include:

- fishy odor, upset stomach or intestines
- increased bleeding, nosebleeds, easy bruising
- increased cholesterol in people with combined hyperlipidemia

- increased caloric intake and weight gain
- added cholesterol in some preparations
- lack vitamin E in some preparations
- concern for oxidation
- vitamin A and D toxicity in some preparations
- pesticide in some fish oils (not highly refined—microfiltered)
- expensive compared to eating fish in the diet

(American Heart Association position, 2001)

Despite the position of the American Heart Association, there is valid reason to consider taking small amounts of fish oils in supplement form. The fact that they contain cholesterol is yet another one of those ridiculous precautions. Also, I don't think we need to worry about the small number of calories you would get from a supplement. First of all, you'd have to eat a lot of fish oil before it could make you fat! Secondly, the whole point of taking fish oil would be to use that good fat as building blocks for key molecules in the body. In fact, fish oils are a good source of two important fatty acids: eicosapentaenoic (EPA) and docosahexaenoic acids (DHA). Fish oil supplementation should be a major consideration during pregnancy, breast-feeding and the early years of a child's life for many reasons. ADHD management should most definitely include fish oil supplementation. It is important that the source of fish oil supplementation you choose is micro-filtered. To be further proactive about your health, you can also request that the manufacturer provide research to show that it is bioavailable. Consumer demand is often the best initiative for food suppliers and supplement manufacturers to provide more valuable information about their products. So use your power.

It looks very promising, especially for those of us with a genetic predisposition for heart disease, that a diet balanced with omega-3 fatty acids may help prevent the biggest health risk facing most Americans. There is also much evidence to show that omega-3 fatty acids can protect the brain as well. Essential fatty acids are the precursors for the synthesis of longer poly-unsaturated fatty acids such as EPA and DHA. The brain is particularly rich in poly-unsaturated fatty acids, such as DHA. If mice are fed a diet including fish oil, which is rich in DHA, the DHA is quickly incorporated into the membranes of their brain cells (Suzuki et al., 1997). Furthermore, brain tissue degradation is correlated to a loss of DHA concentrations. Any treatment related to brain function, such as ADHD and depression, should most definitely include supplementation with DHA. Again, aging is related to oxidative damage to susceptible poly-unsaturated fatty acids; and neurodegenerative disorders, such as Parkinson's and Alzheimer's disease, also appear to exhibit membrane loss of poly-unsaturated fatty acids. So, it is highly possible that if we subscribe to an optimal diet that includes a balance of omega-6 and omega-3 fatty acids, this may help to delay the onset of neurodegenerative disorders (Das, 2000; Youdim et al., 2000).

This is a fertile area of research, and many questions remain to be answered. Whether you choose to supplement or not, I would add that cod liver oil is not a good source of fish oil supplementation, since it might lead to an overdose of vitamin A. For now, I choose to eat lots of wild fish. In general, my diet also consists of a variety of whole foods that contain balanced fats, such as nuts and seeds. One caution here is that often when people hear the recommendation to eat more dietary fat, they go to the extreme and start eating excessive amounts of butter, cream, nuts and other calorie-dense fats. A little bit is beneficial, whereas too much is too much. So, given a daily diet of 1,800–2,000 total calories, fat should make up about 30% of those calories. This is about 4–5 tablespoons or 60–70 grams of fat. To be sure you get a variety of fats in your diet, you might try the following sample menu:

- 2 eggs cooked in a non-stick pan with 1/2 tablespoon of butter for breakfast
- 1 tablespoon of flaxseed oil as part of a salad dressing at lunch
- 2–3 grams of fish oil in supplement form
- 1 tablespoon of olive oil over vegetables, or a lean meat dish at dinner

I supplement my daily diet with 3–4 grams of essential fats from a variety of sources:

- flaxseed oil
- borage oil
- micro-filtered fish oil (from wild fish, like salmon, a good source of the two important omega-3 fats, EPA and DHA)
- soy lecithin
- flax seeds
- wheat germ (which has good fat-soluble vitamins)

Essential fatty acids are now being incorporated into infant formula in some countries. The United States has not caught up yet with adding them in infant formula. Breast milk is rich in poly-unsaturated fatty acids. If you are the parent of an infant and formula is your only option, then I would add about half a teaspoon of flaxseed oil to the formula. But formula is not your only option. Goat milk is a much better alternative to formula as I already discussed in *Chapter Seven*. More people in the world give goat milk to infants and children than any other drink (Haenlein, 1984).

The top of the USDA Food Guide Pyramid shows fats, oils and sweets. These are denoted by symbols that are concentrated in the top of the pyramid and dispersed throughout the other food groups. The USDA suggests that these foods be used sparingly to avoid extra calories. Now that we understand fats a little better, we can see that this category needs to be modified. To be effective, this guide would need to somehow differentiate between helpful unsaturated fats and harmful damaged fats. The USDA Food Guide Pyramid Booklet has my permission to use this helpful overview.

A Quick Guide to Harmful and Helpful Fats

- **Completely cut out trans fats.** Avoid all foods that say, "partially-hydrogenated fat." Remember that food companies keep changing terminology in trying to stay one step ahead of consumer awareness. So be cautious of any packaged food with vegetable oil in it, especially if it has a long shelf life at room temperature. The manufacturer should go out of its way to make it clear to you that the fat in its product is OK, by using words like "no trans fat" and "store in the refrigerator."
- **Avoid cooking with fat.** If this one is difficult for you, then at least use low heat and small amounts of saturated fats, such as butter or coconut oil. A second choice would be to use mono-unsaturated fats, such as olive oil.

- **Include omega-3 fatty acids along with other poly-unsaturated fats in our diet.** This can be done with supplementation and by eating wild fish, grass-fed meat, and omega-3 rich eggs[8].
- **Protect poly-unsaturated fatty acids with the power of antioxidants, such as vitamin E and lecithin.** Vitamin E can be found in whole foods such as leafy green vegetables, almonds, hazelnuts, meat, poultry, fish and in whole food based supplements, such as Juice Plus+®. In fact, Juice Plus+® has been clinically shown to protect fats, as I explained in *Chapter Eight.* Lecithin can be found in soy lecithin granules (available in the refrigerated section of your health food store).

I've shared my best recommendations based on the information available today. But it's important to realize that research is ongoing and new ideas will emerge everyday. It is exciting to me that some researchers are choosing to focus on how to supplement the original Stone Age diet, in order to meet the modern challenge of a growing population that is living longer than our ancestral counterparts. That is, cave dwellers didn't have to worry about aging gracefully. They were lucky if they escaped the hazards of weather, predators and microbes, and made it past 30 years of age.

An anti-aging, fat supplement available on the market today is called "SuperGLA/DHA." It was developed in response to the discovery that as we age, our ability to make an important enzyme called delta-6-desaturase (D6D) decreases. This decline in D6D function inhibits the synthesis of two important fatty acids, gamma-linolenic acid

---

[8] Organic eggs are not necessarily omega-3 rich. Consider the food chain. If the chickens aren't allowed to roam freely, then they are only eating the grains being fed to them. They need to be purposely fed omega-3 fats or at least eat natural vegetation in order to produce eggs that have a balanced ratio of omega-3 to omega-6 fatty acids.

(GLA) from LA, and DHA from LNA. Another critical effect on the body is that several hormones that have important anti-inflammatory and immunoregulatory effects fall out of homeostasis. The reduced capacity to make GLA and DHA as we age is associated with conditions such as:

- cardiovascular disease
- diabetes
- alcoholism
- atopic dermatitis
- premenstrual syndrome
- rheumatoid arthritis
- cancer
- learning deficits
- the development of dementia

(Bolton-Smith et al., 1997; Horrobin, 1993; Jordan, 2001)

Supplementation with GLA and DHA can circumvent impaired D6D function; furthermore, GLA supplementation actually increases D6D function in animal studies (Biagi et al., 1991). You can find this SuperGLA/DHA supplement on the Web at www.lef.org. But I always take less than what is recommended on essential oil supplement bottles. Instead, I choose a variety of sources every day.

Myth #5: Carbohydrates are not fattening.

All carbohydrates (vegetables, fruits, bread, pasta, rice, chips, crackers, desserts, juice, table sugar, etc.) eventually get broken down into a simple sugar called "glucose," which is the currency of choice for the body's energy needs. When we talk about blood sugar levels, we are referring to glucose levels in the blood. Glucose can be used up for energy by our cells; or glucose molecules are strung together in a chain, by the action of enzymes, to make glycogen molecules as a way to store energy; or glucose can be converted into fat for storage of energy as well. Glycogen is stored in your muscles and in your liver. The liver keeps close tabs on glycogen because your brain is always hungry for sugar (glucose) and it's the liver's job to see that your brain gets that sugar. The carbohydrates that are most beneficial to us are the ones that contain fiber and other micronutrients; these would be vegetables, fruits and, I say with caution, whole grains. I am tentative about mentioning whole grains because people often interpret this to mean that it is OK to eat bread, pasta and rice. But many of these foods come in processed forms, and this makes them "incomplete" carbohydrates.

Incomplete carbohydrates are processed carbohydrates. The processing generally removes fiber and important micronutrients. This has several important consequences because these incomplete carbohydrates:

- can raise blood sugar too quickly
- are more likely get stored as fat in the body
- increase the free radical load in the body because they lack sufficient micronutrients

For the purpose of this discussion, I'll use the words "carbohydrate" and "sugar" interchangeably. Also, remember that all carbohydrates can be broken down or converted into glucose—the simple sugar that is directly used for energy by all our cells. When we eat more carbohydrates than we can readily burn for energy, then the excess glucose is either stored as glycogen or converted to fat. Glycogen storage is always helpful to the body. Because we have a limited amount of storage space for glycogen, we can't overdo it. On the other hand, fat storage seems to have no limit. Thus, fat storage, in excess, can be harmful. Glycogen stores greatly increase the amount of energy we have available to us between meals and during exercise. For example, an average 150-pound man has only about 60 calories worth of glucose circulating in his blood, which he can use up in about one hour of sleeping; but he has more than 1,600 calories worth of energy stored in the form of glycogen (Stryer, 1988). The body depends on this stored glycogen. Without it we'd never get to take a break from eating. That 60 calories worth of glucose wouldn't last very long with our active lifestyles. And even thinking requires energy. The hypothalamus part of the brain constantly monitors how much glycogen is available in your liver because the liver is the store where your brain shops for the energy it needs in order to function. Run out of glycogen and you'll experience hunger, followed by a sugar crash.

Unfortunately, simply eating a lot of carbohydrates doesn't maximize glycogen stores because not all excess carbohydrates get converted to glycogen. Some of the excess sugar in the body gets converted to fat. Why? One reason is that we have a limited capacity for storing carbohydrates in the form of glycogen, whereas, in case you haven't noticed yet, we seem to have an infinite capacity to store fat! Another reason we convert excess sugars into fat has to do with the poor choice of carbohydrates in the typical diet. We seem to be attracted to incomplete carbohydrates that do not have a sufficient amount of fiber. When these incomplete carbohydrates break down to glucose, there is not enough fiber present to slow down the entry of that glucose into the blood stream. This allows blood sugar to rise too quickly, which, in turn, signals the body to secrete insulin to help reestablish normal blood glucose levels. In order for normalization to take place as quickly as possible, insulin signals for the excess glucose to be converted into fat, as well as glycogen. In fact, during blood sugar spikes (times when blood sugar is particularly high), fat storage can begin long before glycogen stores become full.

So let's take a look at what happens to the man in the example above, who, as you'll remember, weighs 150 pounds and can store up to 1,600 calories in the form of glycogen. Consider that at the time he chooses to have his next meal, his glycogen stores have come down to about 1,000 calories. So, when he eats a meal with 1,000 calories worth of carbohydrates, only a maximum of 600 calories from carbohydrates can be stored as glycogen. When he then goes home and sits down in front of the television, only a small amount of the carbohydrate calories will be used up for energy. The rest of the carbohydrate calories he ate will get turned into fat.

Furthermore, if the carbohydrates he ate were pasta and bread, then the sugar would enter his blood more quickly and prompt his body to secrete a large dose of insulin. This in turn would promote a faster conversion of the eaten carbohydrates into storable fats. In other words, he would make things even worse by not even filling his glycogen stores before he has started to turn his pasta and bread into body fat. The problem with stimulating unnecessary fat storage is that the body has a general resistance to using that fat later as an energy source. We like to hang on to fat as long as possible, perhaps because, not unlike our Stone Age ancestors, we always seem to be preparing for a famine.

The carbohydrate foods that cause a glucose spike and promote more fat storage are described as carbohydrates with a high glycemic index. The glycemic index is an important measure of the speed at which various carbohydrates can be converted by the body into simple sugars that can enter, and be detected in, the bloodstream. The glycemic index is measured relative to glucose, which is set at a glycemic index of 100. Again, it's not simply the grams or calories of carbohydrate that are so important—but rather the glycemic index, which plays a big role in hormone homeostasis. Such a measure allows us to learn a great deal about the quality of the food that we eat, and hopefully that knowledge will, in turn, help us to make dietary choices that are truly helpful to the body.

Many factors determine this glycemic index.

- The presence of fat in the meal will lower the glycemic index. So, from a purely glycemic index point of view, it is better to eat a piece of toast with butter, as opposed to a dry piece of toast. But, just to be clear, my recommendation is still not to eat bread.
- The presence of protein in the meal will lower the glycemic index. Eating a few eggs with the toast will help much more.
- The type of simple sugar in the food—for instance fructose in fruit has to be converted into glucose; thus the conversion time lowers the glycemic index.

- The type of complex sugar—for instance lactose in milk—has to be broken down into glucose and galactose and the galactose then has to be converted into glucose; all this chemical processing lowers the glycemic index.
- The presence of fiber physically slows down the entry of glucose into the blood.

The best carbohydrates are the ones with lots of fiber. What is so special about fiber? Fiber is a matrix of sugar molecules (called cellulose) found only in plants. But the body does not convert fiber into sugar and use it as a source of energy. In contrast, starch is another example of a sugar matrix found in plants that the body does break down as a source of energy. The reason the body converts starch, but not fiber, hinges on its capacity to make the respective enzymes needed for the breakdown process. The enzyme "cellulase" breaks down cellulose fibers into simpler sugar molecules, whereas amylase breaks down starch. Amylase is present in saliva and can break down starch, but the body never makes cellulase and, therefore, cannot break down cellulose fibers. Even though the body cannot digest fibers for energy, this bulky matrix actually serves our health in other ways.

There are two types of fibers: soluble and insoluble. Soluble fibers dissolve in water, whereas insoluble fibers do not. We have known about the benefits of fiber for quite some time now. You might think of fiber as a set of cleaning brushes for your insides. The soluble fibers keep the blood stream clean, and the insoluble fibers keep the gastrointestinal tract clean. Soluble fiber also helps regulate blood sugar, e.g., the pectin fibers found in the whites of oranges and skin of apples.

Soluble Fibers	Found in
Pectins	Fruits (apples, strawberries, citrus fruits)
Beta-glucans	Oats, barley
Gums	Beans, cereals (oats, rice, barley), seeds, seaweed
Insoluble Fibers	**Found in**
Cellulose	Leafy vegetables such as cabbage, root vegetables such as carrots and beets, bran, whole wheat, beans
Hemicellulose	Skin of seeds and grains
Lignin	Plant stems, leaves and skin (freshly ground flax seeds are a good source)

(Rinzler, 1999)

Carbohydrates such as fruits and, especially, vegetables have a higher fiber content naturally and this fiber content serves to reduce their glycemic indices. The lower amount of fiber in other sources of carbohydrates, such as most breads and pastas, is a factor in their higher glycemic index. That means calorie for calorie, the body converts bread and pasta into body fat much, much more easily than it does vegetables and fruits. In fact, you would have to eat inordinate amounts of vegetables and fruits, in their raw form with fiber present, before the body would convert those calories into fat.

Yet, the USDA Food Guide Pyramid suggests that we eat 6–11 servings of breads, cereals, rice and pastas per day—without making the distinction that refined carbohydrates are high on the glycemic index and, therefore, should be avoided as much as possible. A recently published study suggests that this USDA Food Guide Pyramid needs serious revision. This study included 75,521 women, between the ages of 38–63 years, with no previous diagnosis of diabetes mellitus, myocardial infarction, angina, stroke, or other cardiovascular diseases when the study began in 1984. Researchers followed the women's diets for 10 years and concluded that a diet of refined carbohydrates with a high glycemic index increases the risk of heart disease, independent of previous risk factors (Liu et al., 2000).

High glycemic index foods also give us a false sense of hunger even though we actually have plenty of energy reserves. This is due to the large fluctuations of blood glucose levels that follow a meal high in these carbohydrates. First, there is a glucose surge, which leads to the secretion of insulin. Then there is a drop, as blood sugars are being converted into fat and glycogen by the action of insulin. The liver detects this drop in blood sugar; but because of the presence of insulin, a storage hormone, the liver does not release sugar from glycogen stores. Instead, the liver sends a signal to the hypothalamus part of the brain to go ahead and eat some more food in order to reestablish blood sugar levels. Of course, at this point, the foods we crave will be high in sugar. A review of the current research shows that indeed high glycemic index carbohydrates tend to cause overeating behaviors (Roberts, 2000). These foods can also increase our susceptibility to stress, and we'll discuss this relationship in a later chapter.

Myth #6: A vegetarian diet is a healthy diet.

Proteins such as red meats have had a bad reputation with some people, mostly because they can often contain unbalanced or damaged fats. For example, if a serving of meat has a lot of poly-unsaturated fat in it, and we overcook it, most of that fat will get damaged in the process.

Furthermore, we discussed that the omega-3 and omega-6 fat ratios may be totally off, depending on what the animal or fish or bird has had in its diet. But lean protein, minus the fat complications, is still required in our diets if the body is to make all the enzymes that it needs to function.

In order to understand the value of protein, we need to understand the value and function of enzymes. The body breaks down the protein we eat into amino acids, which then serve as the building blocks for the various enzymes that activate the functions of the body. *Enzymes are protein molecules that have catalytic properties.* We have talked quite a bit about enzymes as the catalysts that make all the chemical reactions in the body go forward. None of the chemical reactions that occur in the body would happen on their own without the help of enzymes. So we would not be able to think, breathe, see, eat or pump blood without enzymes. Enzymes perform their invaluable role by creating favorable nooks and crannies within themselves in which chemical reactions can take place. So, the three-dimensional structure of an enzyme is critical if the enzyme is to be able to act as a catalyst. Most enzymes in the body are short-lived, because they have a hard time maintaining their three-dimensional structure in the milieu of chemical activity occurring in a cell. Once they lose their shape, these enzymes get degraded. If we want the body to work optimally, it is our job to select foods that will constantly replenish the active enzyme pool.

Enzymes are made up 20 amino acids, and 9 of these are essential amino acids that we must get from our diet. Thus, in order for the body to function properly, we need to eat some protein all the time. While many foods contain protein, only some are considered "complete protein" sources. There are two important questions that must be addressed when selecting a complete protein source.

- Can we *absorb* the protein from that food?
- Does that protein contain all of the essential amino acids?

What is considered to be a complete protein has confused many vegetarians. Like it or not, animal protein—dairy, eggs, meat, fish and poultry—are the ideal sources of protein. They are complete because they provide essential trace minerals that are not found in vegetable sources, not even in lentils and beans. Even tofu is missing key minerals. For instance, zinc is critical to the development of the brain and nervous system, and for maintaining the immune system. Zinc deficiency, however, is common among strict vegetarians and can cause a "spacey" feeling that some vegetarians may mistake for a "high from spiritual enlightenment" (Fallon and Enig, 2000). And, zinc supplements are not necessarily a good answer for the reasons that we already discussed in *Chapter Nine*.

Vegetarians are also in danger of missing out on key nutrients like vitamin B_{12}, which is not found in plants. Some vegetarian authorities claim that certain fermenting bacteria in the intestines produce B_{12}. While this may be true, it is in a form unusable by the body. Since B_{12} requires an intrinsic factor from the stomach for proper absorption in the small intestine, the body doesn't absorb the B_{12} made by intestinal bacteria because it doesn't have this intrinsic factor (Byrnes, 2001).

Vitamin B$_{12}$ deficiency is especially a problem for vegans who eat no animal products at all. I've always been perplexed by the vegans who live in certain parts of India and don't suffer from vitamin B$_{12}$ deficiency. Like other people interested in the field of nutrition, I wondered if plant foods do provide vitamin B$_{12}$ after all. Then researchers realized that many small insects, their eggs, larvae and the residue from larvae are left on the plant foods that these people consume, due to fact that they don't use pesticides or have cleaning methods that make their food completely sterile. This, then, is how these people obtain their vitamin B$_{12}$. Researchers noticed that Indian Hindus who are vegans come down with megaloblastic anaemia within a few years after migrating to places like England. They then realized that in England, the food supply is cleaner, and insect residues are completely removed from plant foods (Ibid). So, living a long life means eating meat—whether it's fish meat, bird meat, animal meat or bug meat. You get to choose. I won't look. In fact, I wonder if there is such a thing as a "true herbivore." Is it actually possible for an animal to munch on vegetation and still somehow avoid the bugs, their eggs, their larvae and the larvae residue? In the dictionary it says that an herbivore is "an animal that feeds *chiefly* on plants." It doesn't say "*solely* on plants."

While I sincerely advise against a totally plant-based diet, vegetarianism is sometimes a good choice for cleansing the body. Several health conditions, such as gout for instance, can often be improved by a temporary reduction in animal products with an increase of plant foods. But vegetarianism is not a suitable lifelong practice. Like it or not, humans are a part of the food chain and there are vital nutrients found only in animal products that we must ingest for optimal health. For further reading, I suggest an excellent article by Stephen Byrnes, Ph.D., titled *The Myths of Vegetarianism*. (See *Suggested Reading*, page 343.)

Vegetarian or not, most people tend to eat a diet high in processed carbohydrates and low in sufficient good fats and protein. In the absence of sufficient protein, the body is forced to go into emergency mode and choose to maintain the most vital organs at the expense of other organs. Usually the body will choose to preserve the heart first, but sometimes preserving the brain will take precedence. The body will cannibalize other tissue protein for the amino acid building blocks it needs in order to keep the heart and brain going. Extreme atrophy of other tissues can occur with prolonged starvation, as is seen with anorexia patients. Other organs can deteriorate to the point of no return where death becomes inevitable. For most people, a lack in protein means a less than optimally functioning mind and body, and a slower weakening of both over time. This more gradual decline is referred to as sarcopenia. Sarcowhat? We'll answer that question in the next chapter.

By now, you've begun to appreciate the many negative effects of the Default Health Program diet.

- We've been buying too many products that say "no fat," "low fat," and "no cholesterol."
- We've been eating too many processed foods that are high on the glycemic index and contain damaged fats such as the often-considered-healthy cracker (sugar + trans fat, yum!).

• We've not been eating enough essential fatty acids.
• We've not been eating enough disease-fighting, lean-body producing vegetables and fruits.
• We've not been eating sufficient wild, lean, animal protein with its unique source of vitamins and minerals.

The Longevity Pyramid

While the Default Health Program includes a diet with too many high glycemic index foods, the wrong fats, and not enough of the good fats, protein, and vegetables and fruits, when people try to eat better by following the USDA Food Guide Pyramid, things don't improve much. What the body really needs is a Stone Age diet. As we've learned, the pre-agricultural diet of lean meat, fish, vegetables, fruits and nuts that were foraged from the land has shaped our modern nutritional needs. For optimal gene expression to take place, we need to adopt a diet to fit our genes. Cereals were introduced only 10,000 years ago—during the Agricultural Revolution. Prior to this, humans ate a wide variety of plants. Today, 90% of the world's food supply comes from only about 17% of the available plant species. Three cereals, wheat, maize and rice, account for 75% of the world's grain production, and there is no precedent in human history for such large-scale consumption of what are essentially grass seeds (Papas, 1999). Furthermore, these foods are low in phytonutrients and fiber as compared to vegetables and fruits.

Are you beginning to wonder if perhaps you've been buying too many refined carbohydrates from the isles of the grocery store? It has to be obvious by now that these refined carbohydrates are not helping your body. What to do? If you want to optimize your health, start picking and gathering your

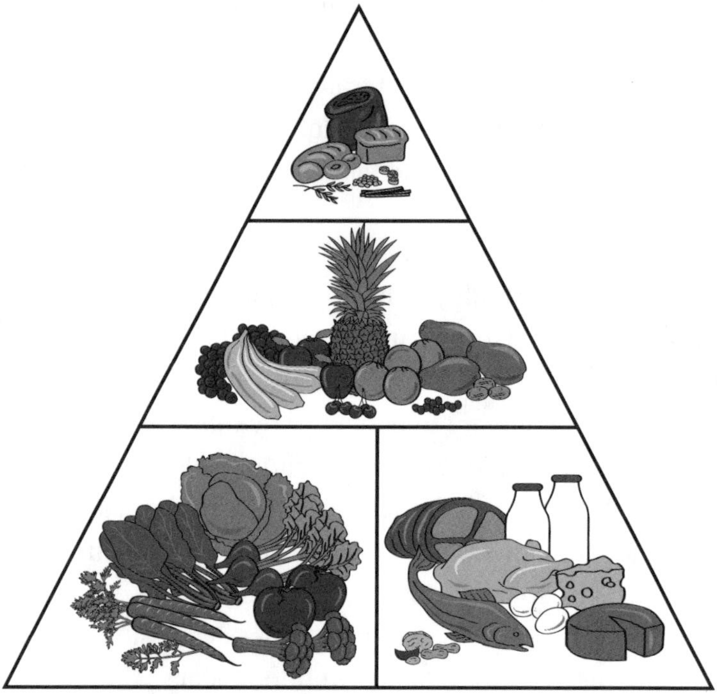

Food Group	Servings	Foods
Grains, breads and cereals	Maximum 2 (0 servings for those interested in losing weight)	Sprouted breads, high-fiber, old-grain cereals and pasta or brown rice
Fruits	2–4	Include many colors, skin and other fibers as possible
Non-starchy vegetables	5–10 ½ cup each	Include many colors, raw with essential fatty acids in the dressing or lightly steamed with antioxidant-rich curries
Meat, fish and poultry	2–3	Wild fish, free-range meat or poultry
	1	Organic milk or cheese
	1	Lentils or beans; a small handful of raw nuts or seeds

Figure 21. The Longevity Pyramid

carbohydrates in the produce isle. If you still crave rice, pasta or cereal, *limit your intake* and choose from the following:

- organic brown rice
- pastas and cereals made from more ancient grains such as spelt, kamut and amaranth, which have more fiber and other essential nutrients

If you are craving bread, my first instinct is to say "Tough it out!" But the kinder, gentler me relents and says, "Oh, all right. Every once in a while you can get away with one of these":

- breads from sprouted grains (usually found in the refrigerated section of health food stores)
- home-baked bread, made with butter

Definitely avoid buying any bread with partially hydrogenated fats (any bread that can sit at room temperature for days without rotting probably has trans fats in them).

Each meal we eat should have some complete protein in it. The average person requires anywhere from 40–70 grams of protein. How much protein is needed partly depends on size, physical activity level and general state of health. Without going crazy and measuring out every portion, you can check out the size of the palm of your hand and use that to estimate the absolute maximum size of the piece of fish, chicken or other lean meat that you should have at any one meal. If you can't hold it in the palm of your hand, then it's too much. On the other hand, there should be some amount of protein in your hand. Other options for meeting your daily protein requirement include eggs, plain yogurt, and other dairy products. I hope that you'll soon be experiencing the benefits of a diet based on the new Longevity Pyramid. *It's not enough to dispel old myths; we have to be willing to live new truths.* Eating right should be fairly simple, and it shouldn't require measuring every gram of food that we eat. Nor should eating right require that we carry an elaborate list of good foods vs. bad foods (based on blood type or some other new fad diet) with us to the grocery store. Dieting or forcing oneself to eat less should also be unnecessary—if we eat the right foods in the right proportions. Once the body has received the nutrients it needs to function, there should be a natural curbing of the appetite. If we'll take just a moment to listen before we take that second helping, hopefully the body will be telling us that we've already given it all of the nutrients it needs in order to maintain or regain health.

Of course, when we introduce these new eating habits, there may be a detoxification period. This incredibly beneficial process may have some seemingly negative, albeit short-term, side effects. The immune system and the digestive system are the primary players involved in detoxification. Let's look at what such efforts to cleanse the body can mean for the person going through detoxification.

- First, when the body finally has enough nutrition to recharge the immune system, it releases immune cells, such as the natural killer cells and other scavenger cells, which can go around and clean up all of the debris that has been accumulating in the body. This important process is similar to the way in which the immune system responds to a viral infection; so, there may be a temporary onset of flu-like symptoms.

- Second, the added nutrition can bolster the activity of friendly bacteria in the gut, and this may mean a short-term increase in gas. This indicates that there has been a change in the process of elimination from the body as rotten food is being flushed from the digestive tract, and as a result, there may be some temporary bloating and gas. You can't imagine how much food is rotting in the nooks and crannies of your intestines in the absence of fiber-rich vegetables.

Detoxification can also mean a drop in hormone levels as the body returns to homeostasis. If serotonin levels drop, you may feel tired or depressed during detoxification; but once you've passed this unpleasant phase, you should start to feel better than you have in years. And it should be relatively simple to stay on track, without feeling like you're depriving yourself of eating a good, hearty meal. If you're still tempted to continue to eat according to the USDA Food Guide Pyramid, I can guarantee that you will always struggle with your weight. In the next chapter we'll discuss the finer points—the "how and when"—of eating from the new Longevity Pyramid.

12

Sarcowhat?

When we're young, life is spread out before us like an all-you-can-eat buffet. We seem to have infinite possibilities and plenty of time. Only when we grow older does it gradually dawn on us that we're not immortal after all and that life necessarily involves choices. We can't continue to eat everything on the buffet—and still remain healthy. Another startling realization is that the body starts to wither as we age. Unless there is intervention, muscles, organs, ligaments and bones become weaker and fat cells become larger. This disgusting process has an official name: *sarcopenia*. The term comes from the Greek roots "sarco," meaning "flesh," and "penia," meaning "reduction in amount or need." I just think of it as the aging of our flesh.

Derivation aside, the most important thing we need to know about sarcopenia is that this process can be slowed down—and even reversed. There are many contributing factors that are actually within our control. In this chapter, we'll discuss the most important of these; I'll implicate the toxic food environment, lack of exercise and ongoing stress for the role that each plays in this premature aging process. The resulting loss of bone density that can accompany sarcopenia is what modern medicine refers to as osteoporosis. Once you understand the many factors that contribute to overall loss of flesh and bone, you'll understand why osteoporosis treatment with calcium supplements is over-simplistic and ineffective. Similarly, the treatment of any degenerative disease with one or a handful of pharmaceutical chemicals misses the mark if it doesn't also address the causes of sarcopenia.

How many people do you know who spend each and every day suffering with backaches and sore joints and, at the same time, accept it as a necessary part of growing old? I'd like to reassure you from the outset that debilitating sarcopenia is not an inevitable part of aging. And here's some more good news: it's a myth to think that you can't build muscle mass well into your nineties. This exciting revelation comes from over a decade of research done at Tufts University. For instance, in one eight-week study, 87- to 96-year-old women who had previously been confined to a nursing home showed that resistance exercise tripled muscle strength and increased muscle size by 10% (Evans and Rosenberg, 1992).

Exciting news, you say, but what does muscle mass have to do with sarcopenia? Well, the one word answer is "everything." That is, if we want to understand sarcopenia, we must first understand the concept of "muscle mass" or "lean mass." Lean mass is the machinery that is our body—our muscles, our organs, our ligaments and connective tissue, our skin, our bones and basically everything else that is not fat tissue. Lean mass is rich in enzymes that carry out the vital chemical reactions that make our body function. Because the research related to body composition has been done mainly on muscle tissue, much of the literature only uses the term "muscle mass." However, in most cases, what is really meant by the term "muscle mass" is "lean mass," which includes our organs and bones. As we age, the loss of lean mass results in lower vitality. It's not just our muscles that get weak, but often our organs and bones as well.

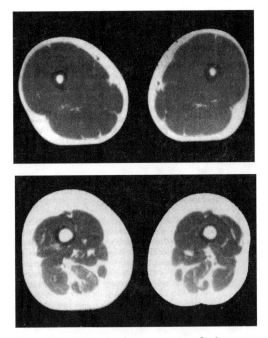

Figure 22. Proportion of lean body mass versus fat in young and older women. These two magnetic resonance images make a dramatic point about the loss of lean body mass and the accumulation of fat as we age. Both show a cross-sectional view of a woman's thigh. The top photo is the thigh of a 20-year-old athlete with a Body Mass Index [BMI] of 22.6. The bottom one is the thigh of a sedentary 64-year-old woman with a BMI of 30.7. Reprinted with permission of Simon & Schuster from BIOMARKERS by William Evans, Ph.D. and Irwin H. Rosenberg, M.D. Copyright ©1991 by Dr. Irwin H. Rosenberg, Dr. William J. Evans and Jacqueline Thompson.

Meanwhile, fatty tissue increases in volume. This is clearly seen in *Figure 22*, which compares the respective cross-sections of two women's thighs. One is that of a 20-year-old athlete, while the other is that of a 64-year-old, sedentary woman. If we were to look at these thighs from the *outside*, we might think that the older woman looks good, because the circumference of her thigh is the same as that of a fit 20-year-old. Interestingly, the 64-year-old woman would weigh less on a scale than the 20-year-old would, and nobody would guess from her appearance that old age had made her fatter. Yet what is going on *inside* tells a completely different story. The 64-year-old woman has hardly any muscle tissue left.

While most people may not know the term sarcopenia, they do think that it's inevitable that their muscles and bones will get weaker with age. This belief is simply a myth that appears real because sarcopenia is the most prevalent end result of the Default Health Program. The problem with sarcopenia is that it's not just a matter of your weight or your physical appearance. You could be suffering unnecessarily from sarcopenia without realizing it. Here is a list of just a few of the symptoms that accompany a loss of lean mass (Ibid., 1992):

- weakness
- less aerobic capacity
- insulin resistance
- high blood pressure
- osteoporosis
- inability to maintain body temperature

Sarcopenia and the immune system

There is an important relationship between a properly functioning immune system and our ability to maintain lean body mass. Many people, especially athletes and individuals under a lot of emotional stress, don't appreciate this connection and have a hard time avoiding every cold or flu that comes around. It's true that we can do almost nothing to keep microbes from entering the body, but if microbe exposure is kept to a low level and remains fairly constant, it can actually serve to challenge and strengthen the body's immune system (Zinkernagel, 2001). At the same time, we also need to safeguard the immune system. When we catch a bug, instead of purchasing pharmaceuticals and/or pushing ourselves to keep working, the best thing we can do is rest. Really? Yes, really! When the immune system is engaged in making antibodies and immune cells, such as natural killer cells, it uses extra energy and lots of nutrients from the body—amino acids to make the needed antibodies, and all the components needed to make new immune cells. Instead of fighting this process by trying to continue with our hectic schedules, it's important to rest, so that the immune system can have all of the resources it needs to fight disease. And remember, when you're resting, you're not just killing time. Your natural killer cells are hard at work. Help your immune system to do its job, and it will develop a powerful memory of the bug that you've contracted and be better able to recognize and deal with it in the future. Pharmaceuticals, on the other hand, while alleviating some symptoms, will most likely hinder this process.

We can appreciate just how much the immune system depends on the body's resources by looking at the way in which lean mass can atrophy during long periods of illness. I'll share with you my own experience of this. When I was eleven, I went back to India for a visit. While I was there, I came down with typhoid fever. Yes, I had received a typhoid vaccination before the trip; I got sick nonetheless. To make matters worse, I proved to be allergic to the antibiotics that were the accepted treatment; so in the end, it was probably my immune system's proper response both to the memory of the vaccination, as well as to the real microbe itself that saved my life. I was a skinny kid to begin with and, after a week in bed with a strong fever, I reportedly lost 15 pounds. The important point is that I survived. Studies with critically ill children have shown that there is a huge increase in protein turnover, a decrease in the synthesis of proteins, and a reprioritizing in favor of the proteins that are crucial to survival (Curley and Castillo, 1998). So, my lean mass served as the reservoir from which my immune system could tap in order to fight the organism that had moved into my body.

It may seem as if I'm suggesting that someone should have been giving me large meals of protein while I was ill, but this would not have been helpful either. When we get sick, digestion becomes an exhaustive task, drawing energy and resources away from the immune system for the making of digestive enzymes. When we get sick from a microbe, one of the most important things to do is to rest and to eat light meals that are easy to digest; this will minimize recovery time and loss of lean mass.

Such a loss of lean mass can also occur as we gradually age and the immune system becomes more dysfunctional through DNA mutations. As we discussed before, a diet lacking in antioxidant-rich vegetables and fruits weakens the immune system, which can start making unnecessary antibodies. This, in turn, can often lead to autoimmune disorders, where the body starts to make antibodies to itself. The other consequence of a weakened immune system is that it becomes inefficient at responding to invading microbes. To lower our chances of getting sick, it's very important to maintain a good diet that supports the immune system at all times with adequate micronutrients and macronutrients. During illness, it's critical to minimize any competition with our immune system for essential nutrients. I can't emphasize enough that rest is critical for recovery and for minimizing any loss of lean mass.

Building lean mass

Macronutrients can be used to make lean body mass or body fat. Which would you prefer? Well, it's not that easy. There are hormones that regulate that choice. Growth hormone is responsible for growth of lean mass, while insulin is responsible for energy storage. An interesting fact about growth hormone is that it's secreted according to what is known as a circadian rhythm. The word "circadian" comes from the Latin "circa," meaning "around" and "dies," meaning "day"—in other words, "about a day." As it turns out, our growth hormone secretion peaks during deep sleep. This secretion of growth hormone is especially important for children, because anything that disrupts this normal secretion will slow down their growth. What purpose does growth hormone serve for adults? It serves to rebuild lean mass tissue, and most of this work also gets done while we sleep. Growth hormone secretion has several effects on the body.

- It instructs cells to take up amino acids (the building blocks for enzymes) circulating in the blood in order to synthesize more enzymes.
- It stimulates an increase in the uptake of nutrients needed for the growth of bone and cartilage.
- It mobilizes fat as a source of energy for growth.
- It decreases sugar metabolism and blood sugar.

This circadian rhythm to the release of growth hormone adds an interesting twist to the whole equation—that is, not only do we need to concern ourselves with *what* we eat, but also we need to consider *when* we eat. Since growth requires energy, growth hormone triggers the body to release fat stores, which is opposite to the action of insulin, which is to store fat. Now, one aspect of our default program is that too many of us eat our biggest meal of the day too close to bedtime. When we eat a large meal, blood sugar goes up as we break down our meal. The extra sugar prompts insulin secretion and fat storage. Thus, a late meal has hidden consequences for our health.

- We spend much of our sleep state digesting our meal.
- We increase body fat by the action of insulin.
- We don't release growth hormone when too much insulin is around.
- We don't build lean mass without the aid of growth hormone.

So, eating late meals is a great way to speed up sarcopenia. The converse is also true: if we do most of our eating early in the day, then insulin levels will drop to a minimum during sleep, and the rebuilding of lean mass will be optimized. Another great way to increase the body's natural production of growth hormone is to exercise. While some people try to outsmart the body by supplementing it with growth hormones, these two simple steps—not eating too late at night and exercising—are effective and safe ways to assist the body in maintaining normal growth hormone production.

A word about hormone replacement therapy

Hormone replacement therapy (HRT) is very fashionable today but often inappropriate as a first step. The advertisements for hormone replacement therapies go something like this:

> Hormone X is a naturally occurring substance in the human body that is secreted by the pituitary, the master gland of the body, located in the endocrine system. Hormone X is a microscopic protein substance. Hormone X has all these benefits for the body. Unfortunately, as we age, our production of hormone X goes down. We have a way for you to replace hormone X. Give us a call.

First of all, if you can buy hormone X without a doctor's prescription, other than natural progesterone cream, you can just forget about it. For instance, taking human growth hormone (HGH) in a pill form will do nothing for you; it has to be injected. Even the creams that are prescribed by a physician require repeated testing of the blood in order to monitor hormone levels. Second, people are too quick to run to hormone replacement experts, without first doing all that they can do themselves to reach hormone homeostasis.

Here is some news that might interest you. The pituitary gland is not the "master gland" of the body. Nobel laureates Guillemin and Schally disproved this myth and showed that the brain is the master gland. A specific part of the brain called the hypothalamus is connected to the pituitary by, as my toddler would say, "a teeny, tiny, teeny" little circulatory system which tells the pituitary gland what hormones to make and when. This is very complicated physiology to comprehend and the best minds haven't figured it all out yet. But I want to leave you with what I consider to be the bottom line. The hypothalamus makes its decisions to slow down the production of all those desired hormones such as growth hormone, based on the level of stress you may be experiencing—be it emotional, nutritional or physical stress. So if you are under stress and other key hormones are not in homeostasis, injecting yourself or pumping yourself up with hormones is like trying to burn a candle at both ends.

True, age does diminish the production of these hormones; but the Default Health Program is doing more to subdue desirable hormone levels than age itself. These "youthful" hormones are the luxury of hormone homeostasis. So first, check in with yourself and see if you aren't drawing too much cash from the hormone bank account to begin with before you borrow more money to pay for hormone replacement therapy.

In the next section we'll talk about weight loss. But this discussion isn't limited to people who want to lose weight. The following information is critical for everyone who is interested in longevity.

The myth of weight loss

Perhaps the most prevalent misunderstanding around health has to do with weight loss. These two words have spawned a subculture, a whole new way of life. Enter, the dieters (Homo sapiens sarcowhatitus). They can usually be found:

- drinking diet sodas and eating diet foods
- rubbing lotions and taking potions for those quick "lose 10 pounds in two weeks" plans
- reading endless magazine articles about how the rich and famous lose weight
- comparing themselves to the supermodels or superjocks that have become our role models

This subculture is especially apparent among teenage girls who are scared of the word "fat." But the supermodels that these young girls emulate may be suffering from sarcopenia as much as any fat person on the street.

The bottom line is that weight loss should never be the goal. In reality it's pretty easy to lose weight. You may be saying "What? What about the fact that over half the adult population currently meets the definition of obesity?" Let me explain. The problem is that it's easy to lose the wrong kind of weight. Starve yourself on a low-calorie, low-fat diet and you'll initially lose weight rapidly; but what *kind* of weight will you lose? You'll lose "water weight" and lean mass. This unhealthy form of weight loss can take its toll on your body.

This kind of water weight loss comes from the water

that is released when glycogen molecules are broken down; remember that your body uses glycogen to store the quick energy that is needed for the brain and muscles to function. In the body, stored glycogen is about twice as heavy as stored fat. But just so you're not confused by the term "water weight," here are some hard facts about this glycogen weight:

- Glycogen isn't responsible for making you look plump, bloated or bulky.
- Glycogen doesn't add inches to your waistline.
- Glycogen weight is vital to your health.

For example, your mood, your energy, your cognition, your cravings for sugar are all dependent on your glycogen levels. And since we only store enough glycogen to last for about one day, we need to replenish our stores of glycogen; it's not long-term, like fat storage. Now here is the crux of the confusion around weight loss. I already told you that stored glycogen is about twice as heavy as stored fat. Thus, a 150-pound man with 20 percent body fat would weigh 180 pounds if all of his fat were converted to glycogen. So when the body is deprived of calories, heavy glycogen stores get used up and weight is lost initially, but then suddenly weight loss comes to a halt. Thus, losing "water weight" doesn't really lead to a smaller waistline—it leads to your having less energy, especially for your brain.

Another unhealthy side effect of weight loss is the potential loss of lean mass. Cutting back on food intake, unfortunately, also means cutting back on essential nutrients. This means that lean mass atrophies because there aren't enough nutrients to support it. Furthermore, the brain will break down lean mass protein and convert it into sugar for energy. You will literally be eating yourself in order to save your brain. We discussed this same phenomenon earlier in relation to skipping breakfast. Stored fat (triglycerides) cannot be used for brain energy.

Another problem is that as lean mass goes down, the body's ability to burn fat goes down. This is because it is your lean mass that puts demands on your body fat as a source of fuel in order to do things like maintain body temperature or perform exercise. If the lean mass furnace shrinks, then fat stores can build up more easily. Thus, losing lean mass doesn't make you look any better, and it certainly doesn't improve your health or make you *feel* any better. Think of it this way. Your bones, brain, muscles, and other organs have all lost some of their weight, but those thighs or "love handles" are still there. Meanwhile, you've diminished your ability to burn fat.

Nobody needs to lose "weight," per se. What we should be concerned about is "fat loss." So, you can bet that every weight loss gimmick out there on the market—from diet plans to dangerous herbs and pharmaceuticals—is taking advantage of the fact that it's easy to lose water weight and lean mass. People are so sold on the fluctuation of the needle on their bathroom scale that they don't even know when they're being had. We, as a society, are sold, "hook, line and sinker," on weight loss as a desirable goal. Even after you read this chapter, you may still wake up tomorrow and get on your scale. Most people don't own a stethoscope or a blood pressure monitor. They would probably have to search for a thermometer if asked for one, but they would know exactly where the scale is located. People own scales to tell them something about how they look to other people, and a lower number is always associated with a better look. Don't settle for beauty that's skin-deep. Lean mass can help you radiate the glow of good health that comes from within.

Overweight people are really just suffering from sarcopenia, a condition wherein their lean mass is not large enough to demand more energy from their fat cells. Their fat cells are just too large in size. Yes, that's right, I said "size" not "number" of fat cells. We don't make more fat cells as we age; instead the ones we have just get larger. They know no boundaries. How rude!

What do I mean by saying that the lean mass is not big enough in comparison to the fat? As I mentioned, in order to maintain body temperature, the body is always burning fat, even when we're asleep. The demand on this fat-burning furnace is therefore directly related to how much lean mass we need to keep warm. So the bigger and stronger the lean mass is, the greater its capacity to burn fat. The same is true when you try to exercise your muscles: the more lean mass you have, the more fat you'll need to burn for energy. Thus, increasing lean mass turns out to be the most important way to alter fat metabolism and address sarcopenia. The gimmicks mentioned earlier don't even begin to approach the problem from this angle.

So to anyone wanting to lose weight, I want to say that while there is a fast way to lose weight in terms of water weight and lean mass, there is no quick and easy way to lose fat. A prime example is an eight-week study during which weight-loss patients were given Phen-fen and/or Redux (before they were recalled). The results can be seen in *Figure 23* below.

Note that on a scale, all patients lost weight but all of it was lean mass; more frightening is that 70% gained body fat. A loss in lean mass means a reduction in fat burning capacity. An increase in body fat means that a person will physically look larger and have more health problems. This is the gimmick that sells every diet program that focuses on quick weight loss.

On the other hand, gaining weight could be a good thing. Remember that glycogen is about twice as heavy as fat. Yet having your liver and your muscles full of glycogen is a great thing for your brain and your muscles. Elite athletes try to train their muscles to "carbo load." What they're really trying to do is to maximize their glycogen stores. That way, a long-distance runner has the energy needed to finish that marathon. For our everyday needs, the more glycogen we have, the less our blood sugar fluctuates. And, glycogen

Measurement	% Patient Response
Weight Loss	100%
Lean Mass Loss	100%
Fat Loss	0%
Fat Gain	70%

Figure 23. Body composition after use of diet drugs
(Phen-fen or Redux) (Wise, 1999)

gives ample fuel for the brain to function properly. *We also don't crave processed carbohydrates and stimulants when glycogen stores are full.* So, be mentally prepared; if you take measures to increase your glycogen stores, you may gain some very healthy weight, and the only loss you may see is in your waistline. This is especially evident in people who have body fat percentages below 25%.

Here's where we must really let go of our old ideas about weight loss. *The only healthy and long-term way to lose body fat is to increase your lean mass.* This doesn't necessarily mean an increase on the bathroom scale, but it could. It all depends on how much the lean mass is increasing, and how much the fat is decreasing. Lean mass increases your metabolism and your need to burn fat as a source of fuel. And an increase in lean mass means a subsequent increase in glycogen stores to support that lean mass. So, I recommend that you never try to lose weight too quickly, but, instead, that you prepare yourself for the fact that you may actually *gain* a little weight initially on your way to finally and forever dropping those pounds of fat. The longer you resist this concept and hang on to a desire to find that miracle "quick-loss" plan, the longer the aging process of sarcopenia will control your destiny. End of story.

Don't focus on the weight. Being overweight is *not a disease*; it's only one of the many *symptoms* that tell you that your hormones are out of balance. Since the imbalance of one hormone can lead to an imbalance in many other hormones, it's not always easy to figure out which imbalance came first. But to give you an understanding of the difference between cause and symptom, I've listed three hormone imbalances that can cause "weight gain"—or more accurately, sarcopenia—as well as some accompanying symptoms that may sound all too familiar.

- Blood levels of insulin are too high—a condition called hyperinsulinemia. This can result in "yo-yo" weight gain, cravings for sugar or high glycemic foods, intense hunger, weakness, shakiness, the need for frequent meals, poor concentration, emotional instability, memory disorders, lack of focus, feelings of anxiety and panic, lack of motivation and fatigue.
- Blood levels of glucagon and growth hormone are low. Symptoms may include depression, social isolation, anxiety and low energy.
- Serotonin levels are low, evidenced by depression, fatigue and cravings for processed carbohydrates (bread, pasta, crackers, chips, etc.) and stimulants (alcohol, caffeine and other drugs).

Once you recognize these symptoms and work toward reestablishing hormone homeostasis, the excess fat will begin to melt away. "That sounds like a complicated job," you say, "How do I do that?"

First, I must make a comment about diets that over-compensate for the tendency to eat high glycemic index carbohydrates. These diets are seeking to counter this tendency by recommending a very low amount of carbohydrate intake, especially for the first two weeks, in order to force the body to burn fat as a source of energy. I want to preface my next comments with some personal background information. I am generally a person who dislikes it when reviewers sharply criticize popular books; my take is that if the book is so popular, then there must be something of value, something to learn from it. Maybe I just need to look again in order to see what others are seeing that I'm not. So, please understand that when I'm evaluating the Atkins Diet® (Atkins, 1999) and other such diets, it's not just from an intellectual standpoint, but from having tried it for myself, watching other friends try it, and evaluating and reevaluating what value there might be. In other words, if Dr. Atkins had figured it out, then I'd be one of the first people to jump up and down with joy. My sincere hope is to have people succeed in their goals with reducing their body fat, and even if everyone else in the world were to criticize something, if I sincerely thought that it had merit, I'd share it.

Having said that, the Atkins Diet® and similar diets are also treating all carbohydrates the same; the difference is that the USDA Food Guide Pyramid assumes all carbohydrates are good whereas the Atkins-style diet assumes they are bad for achieving quick weight loss. The USDA Food

Comparison of different carbohydrates
and their ability to release insulin

Food	Total carbohydrates (grams)	Fiber (grams)	Total carbohydrate – fiber = insulin-stimulating carbohydrates (grams)
Pasta (1 cup)	40	2	38
Apple (1 medium)	20	4	16
Raw broccoli (1 cup)	7	4	3

Guide Pyramid touts carbohydrates because they are low-fat foods, failing to take into account that the body can turn them into fat. On the other hand, low carbohydrate diets propagate a generalization that the intake of carbohydrates of any kind will slow down weight loss, because it keeps us from burning body fat. But, I am here to say again, "Hello! *All carbohydrates are not the same.*" Eating 10 grams of chips is not the same as eating 10 grams of broccoli. The chips have empty calories and are high on the glycemic index. Eating chips will cause you to secrete insulin faster, helping to convert those chips into body fat. The broccoli is full of antioxidants that will slow down the aging process; and it's low on the glycemic index, so the sugar will enter your body slowly, supplying your body, especially your brain, with the energy it needs to function.

Well, you probably didn't need me to tell you that you shouldn't be eating chips. But what about the other carbohydrates that we may consider healthy? Did you know, for instance, that soup and pasta are not so good for you? They don't have enough fiber, and they contain more insulin-secreting carbohydrates for about the same volume of food than raw vegetables. Consider the table on the previous page. Notice that for about the same volume of food, there is a large difference in the number of insulin-secreting carbohydrates that these foods contain.

The USDA Food Guide Pyramid and the low-carbohydrate diets are extreme opposites when it comes to their views on carbohydrates. While the body can operate on body fat as a source of energy during a real famine, it is desperate, unpleasant and unnecessary to put the human body through this as a method of weight loss. The health consequences can be enormous. On the other hand, there is some merit in these diets: their recommendation to eat more dietary fat. I totally agree with that aspect, as long as the fats are not damaged fats.

If you should find yourself tempted to try one of these diets that tells you to limit your carbohydrate intake to almost nothing, here are some points to consider about such low carbohydrate diets:

- First, these diets may sound good to some people because you get to eat all kinds of yummy, fatty meats like bacon and sausage. However, these foods contain fats that have been excessively heated and, if they are not organic, may be high in fat-soluble toxins.
- Second, for the sake of your brain alone, it's not good to venture too far into the "omit all carbohydrates camp." The human brain is the biggest sugar-hog around and the hypothalamus is constantly monitoring levels of glycogen in the liver to determine if we should eat or not. If you drastically cut carbohydrates out of your diet, your body will eventually look to fat as a source of energy. You may succeed in forcing your body to burn some fat; but you won't be able to meet your brain's energy needs—it will still need sugar! Your brain cannot use stored fat (triglycerides) as a source of energy. So, you may start to look good in your bikini, but you'll be a dumb "babe" with a bad attitude. And your brain will always crave sugar if your glycogen stores are not full.
- Third, you'll slow down your metabolism on a low carbohydrate diet. Why? Because it triggers an adaptation mechanism that we have retained in order to help us through

periods of famine. Restricting fats or carbohydrates (the two principle macronutrients that give us energy) makes the body think that there is a famine going on. Slowing down your metabolism may have long-term consequences for your ability to stay lean. Remember a naturally faster metabolism usually means a more youthful and desirable metabolism.

• Fourth, a diet limited in carbohydrates is a diet limited in the phytonutrients that come from carbohydrates such as vegetables and fruits; thus you increase your oxidative stress and speed the aging process. These phytonutrients are also critical for protecting the unsaturated fats that we must get in our diets as they keep these fats from going rancid in the body. Dr. Atkins is big on vitamins. He takes hundreds of pills himself; but as I explained in *Chapter Nine*, it's still not enough. It's not whole food.

• Last, these low carbohydrate diets are dehydrating. Raw vegetables and fruits are a great way to increase your intake of water. The volume that veggies and fruits take up is greater per calorie than other foods; and, in addition, hunger can be satiated partially by physically filling up the stomach. Vegetables and fruits also increase your metabolism. Dr. Atkins maintains that his ongoing diet has plenty of vegetables. I beg to differ. Today, no diet has enough vegetables—you almost can't eat the amounts you need to stay healthy because the quality of our produce is suffering from triple cropping and depleted soils. That's why I supplement with Juice Plus+®.

Any plan to reduce body fat must include fiber-rich, phytochemical-rich, antioxidant-rich, mineral-rich, water-rich, metabolism-increasing, low-glycemic index vegetables. It's a considerably more healthy, natural and effective way to go.

My revised plan would be to count only incomplete carbohydrates or man-made carbohydrates and to keep those to a minimum—less than 10 grams a day—while allowing for as many raw vegetables as needed to satiate hunger. A few fruits are OK, too.

Since the Atkins Diet® has been one of the most popular low carbohydrate diets, I'd like to make some additional points that are specific to this diet.

- First, the Atkins Diet® would recommend that in the first couple of weeks you limit carbohydrates to less than 20 grams or so. I say that if you're talking about colas, bread, crackers, cake, cereal, pasta, pretzels and chips, then that is a great idea! In fact, I would lower that amount to less than 10 grams a day or nothing at all, because it's hard to really enjoy 10 or 20 grams of chips and the like. So why do it at all? Ten grams is less than a slice of bread! But, if you're talking about high fiber/low glycemic index vegetables, such as broccoli, cabbage, kale, mixed greens and spinach, then eat them to your heart's content. You can avoid fruit for a few weeks if you really want to give your body a jump-start towards hormone homeostasis; but eat your veggies, even at breakfast.
- Second, while Dr. Atkins tries to distinguish between good fat and bad fat, what I have seen in actual practice is that, for one reason or another, people eat mostly damaged fats when they follow his diet, such as bacon fat. I would recommend eating lean proteins and adding fat that isn't cooked. You should eat 2 tablespoons of good omega-3

fats at every meal.

- Third, I disagree with Dr. Atkins' recommendation to use sugar substitutes, such as aspartame. Stevia is the only sugar substitute that I have no reservations about recommending. Some health food stores sell it in a white powder form, and it's much sweeter than sugar, but with a slightly bitter aftertaste. Stevia is an herb that has been intensely studied and found to have no complications and actually, to have some health benefits. The other option is to just get over your fondness for that sugary taste. As far as your body chemistry is concerned, it only takes three days of concentrated effort to kick the sugar habit cold turkey. Of course, you may still need to deal with other more complicated factors such as the prevalence of sugar in our society and the psychological withdrawal—not a trivial task for most people. (See *Beating Overeating* in *Suggested Reading* for further help on this matter.)
- Fourth, some people start to buy low-sugar snack bars[1], some with the Atkins label. These bars are extremely dehydrating and often contain questionable food additives. When you're trying to get your body to find balance again, it's more important then ever to eat vegetables. Today you can buy pre-cut broccoli, carrots, peppers, etc. and it's no less convenient than a diet bar. You can even buy low-sugar, high-fat, organic salad dressings to dip them in.
- Fifth, limiting carbohydrates to less than 20 grams a day means using up your glycogen stores and losing water weight. So you must keep eating enough veggies so as not to lose glycogen.
- Sixth, it is unhealthy and unnecessary to go into ketosis. Atkins actually recommends that you monitor ketones, a

---

[1] In fact, I don't recommend any bars, since I have yet to find one free of trans fats.

product of fat metabolism, in your urine to make sure that you go into ketosis—burning fat for energy. People who have tried this diet like this part because they can actually monitor something to see if they are being successful. But it's not necessary to urinate on a ketosis stick to know that something is going on; the headache from eliminating processed sugar is enough to let you know that, yes indeed, you are on your way to beating the sugar blues. In fact, what I like about the Atkins Diet® is that when you do drastically reduce your carbohydrate consumption, the body begins to detoxify from the "drug" we are most addicted to as a society—sugar, as William F. Dufty talks about in his book, *Sugar Blues*.

- Finally, there is the reality of the Atkins Diet® and its progression over time. Dr. Atkins himself admits that he doesn't know exactly why the diet works. Perhaps it's presumptuous of me, but I have a pretty good idea why the diet seems to work at least in terms of shifting the bathroom scale to the left. Two things initially occur on his diet. First, the body truly does go into fat burning mode when carbohydrates are kept to less than 20 grams. But this is not a desirable way to lose body fat, especially considering that it's not the only way and that there can be health hazards associated with ketosis. Furthermore, the second thing that happens on this diet is that while most people do see quick weight loss, it's the wrong kind of weight. And, my friends, the only two processes that create quick weight loss are loss of water weight or loss of lean mass. Fat loss is much slower. When all the glycogen stores get depleted after 48 hours of being on a low-carbohydrate diet, a lot of water is released as the chemical bonds that hold glycogen together get broken down. This process is not as productive as it may seem. Losing all that glycogen also means that you've made your brain and muscles very unhappy.

Continuing on this diet does cause weight loss, because when you limit all of those carbohydrates, there's not a lot to choose from; so your caloric intake goes down quite a bit. It ultimately becomes a calorie-restricted diet and not the miraculous, fulfilling diet that it is advertised as being. This has actually been shown in a study using the Atkins Diet®. Subjects in this study went from their usual diet, averaging 2,481 calories per day, to 1,419 calories per day on this diet (Hellmich, 2000).

Ultimately people add back carbohydrates, but with no discretion. They were never taught the importance of the glycemic index. Most people have just been reading a book and not participating in a monitored program; so left on their own, with permission to eat all this fat (greater than 30% of the daily caloric intake), they then add back carbohydrates, such as bread and pasta. This drastically increases caloric consumption and alters hormone balance. Eventually the weight comes back on. Perpetual Atkins dieters I call them, for they must always return to those drastic measures of ketosis over and over again to get back to their desired weight. While Dr. Atkins may think that this is an acceptable practice for life, I think not. Initially, I don't doubt that positive results are seen with serum lipid profiles, blood pressure and other markers of disease when a high carbohydrate diet comes to a halt. But eventually, not being particular about eating good fats and protecting those fats with lots of antioxidant-rich, raw vegetables is going to lead to harm. These dieters were never encouraged to face the reality of the matter: the only diet that works for our genes is the Stone Age diet.

After all of those carefully crafted points to consider, could you *still* be tempted to go on a weight-loss diet? Is there one last gimmick you need to try? Get ready and get real.

> *"We can't solve problems by using the same kind of thinking we used when we created them."*
> —Albert Einstein

This brings me to a point I'd like to make about all the other diet books that you see out there. From where I stand, you will always get some initial results when you follow any kind of plan that has you become aware of what you eat. When we don't monitor what we eat, most of us eat too much; and that in it self is a big problem for all of us. But the only diet that is going to give us a lean body and a long life is the Stone Age diet. So if you can't "hunt it, fish it pick it or milk it," then don't eat it. I know that it sounds like a contradiction to include "milk it" in a Stone Age diet because cave dwellers didn't milk anything. But since infants start life with milk, our genes have "seen" milk for millions of years. So, I think that it's a safe addition to the Longevity Pyramid. Though cave dwellers were probably weaned at no more than four years of age, this is more of a survival issue than a diet issue. Whole, organic cow milk is a balanced meal with complete protein, low-glycemic index carbohydrates, important fats and some key micronutrients. So for those who don't have allergic reactions or digestive problems associated with milk, it does make sense. And while I've given permission to eat butter already, understand that whenever food is processed, you can get into trouble. There is no need to count calories when you are strictly eating whole, unprocessed food. If you start to make cream, butter or cheese from milk, then that's processing, and exercising self-control and calorie counting become important. When you start to make vegetable soup or overcooked vegetable casseroles, then self-control and calorie counting become important. You get the idea. Cave dwellers may not have had any modern luxuries; but at least they could eat without worrying about self-control and calorie counting.

What are you willing to give up doing in order to get what you really want? You'll get the results you want when you give up those images of what you consider to be a great meal. You'll get the results you want when you give up the idea of quick weight loss. You'll get the results that you want when you kick the sugar habit. Here's the program that's going to get you into those tight jeans again. Follow the Ten Rules for Life for two weeks (four weeks for

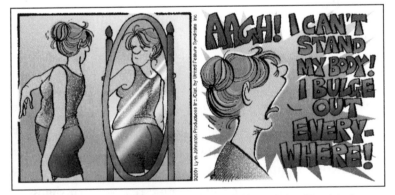

From FOR BETTER OR FOR WORSE ©2001. Reprinted with permission of Lynn Johnston Productions, Inc. All rights reserved. *Reproduced in its entirety in the center of the book.*

extremely stubborn metabolisms) and you will begin to see results. The great thing is that your heart, your brain, your muscles and all your other organs are going to love you for it. Even if you are already an elite athlete, it will make you more elite!

Ten Rules for Life

Rule 1. Eat all of the vegetables you want. Choose a minimum of four different kinds every day. Start your day with veggies and at the end of each week, be sure you've protected yourself with all of the colors of the rainbow. Avoid fruit for these first few weeks. When you do reintroduce fruit, try to have it with a fatty food, such as crème fraiche or heavy cream (unsweetened, of course) and cheese. Eventually you can replace crème fraiche or heavy cream with whole yogurt as an option for the rest of your life.

Rule 2. To make certain vegetables more palatable, lightly steam them and add 1 tablespoon of butter. You can also lightly stir-fry in 1 tablespoon of butter and experiment with a little garam masala spice and a little sea salt. With raw vegetables, use any salad dressing that has no sugar or sugar substitute. Dressings with fat but no sugar or sugar substitutes are OK.

Rule 3. Eat the equivalent of a handful of either free-range eggs, lean meat, poultry or wild fish two to three times a day. Remember, with whole food, it's not about calorie counting; it's about hormone balance. Once your hormones come back to homeostasis, you'll notice that you'll eat less, naturally—as long as you continue to stay

Weight in pounds	Volume of water (ounces)	Volume of water (liters)	Volume of water in 8 oz. glasses
125	84	2.4	10+
150	100	2.8	12+
175	117	3.3	15
200	133	3.8	16+
225	150	4.3	19
250	167	4.7	21
275	183	5.2	23
300	200	5.7	25
325	217	6.1	27

away from man-made carbohydrates. Have at least some protein at every meal, including snacks.

Rule 4. If you couldn't theoretically "hunt it, fish it pick it or milk it," don't eat it. Respect your DNA and remember what Eaton said about the Stone Age diet being the appropriate diet for the proper expression of your genes.

Rule 5. Drink plenty of filtered water in order to facilitate fat loss. Most people don't understand what plenty means. For optimum results, work your way up to drinking 2/3 of your weight in ounces of water (see table on the following page).

Rule 6. Since each meal is limited to only a handful of protein and 1–2 tablespoons of fat, this will automatically limit the amount of food that you can have at any given meal. So, eat five smaller meals a day instead of two or three big meals. Eat more at the beginning and middle of the day, and less at the end of the day. Eat your last meal at least four hours before going to bed in order to improve your quality of sleep. Spreading out your meals will help you eat less overall, while maintaining your energy level and increasing your metabolism.

Rule 7. Supplement your diet as described in the next section.

Rule 8. Exercise (See *Chapter Fourteen*). Exercise will help you build fat-burning lean mass and help you reestablish hormone homeostasis

Rule 9. Manage your stress so that you can get at least seven hours of sleep every night (see *Chapter Thirteen*). Stress releases glucocorticoids, which in turn release insulin, which in turn inhibits fat metabolism and makes you crave carbohydrates. On the other hand, sleeping seven hours allows growth hormone to be released, which in turn allows for making more lean mass.

Rule 10. Measure your percentages of body fat and lean

	JuicePlus+® Test Group	Non-JuicePlus+® Control Group
Fat gain or loss	-5.8 lbs.	-2.5 lbs.
Muscle gain or loss	+1.9 lbs	0.0 lbs.
BCI	+7.7	+2.5

Figure 24. Placebo vs. Set for Life. Subjects were tested after an eight-week trial against placebo. Weight, fat, lean mass and body composition index (BCI) were measured.
BCI = sum of total lean mass increase + body fat decrease.

mass. You can do this at many health clubs or weight loss clinics. Some health care professionals also offer this service. Initially, monitor those percentages every two weeks, instead of weighing yourself every single day. If you absolutely can't find a way to measure your lean mass and body fat, you can monitor your waistline at your belly button and your hip line at its widest point.

Making your life easier

If you're committed to kicking the sugar habit, and you're armed with the knowledge that what you are really fighting is sarcopenia instead of weight loss, it's time for me to share a nutritional program with you. The makers of Juice Plus+® have a complete program designed to increase lean mass and reduce body fat. The program incorporates whole food based supplements (Juice Plus+®), a protein/carbohydrate shake mix (Juice Plus+ Complete®) and fiber wafers (Juice Plus+ Thins®). The combination of these three products (Set for Life) when compared to a placebo group showed a significant increase in lean mass and reduction in body fat. I used to think that strength-training exercise was the only way to significantly increase lean mass and that nutrition only supported that process. But in this study, the subjects were all encouraged to walk more and no strength-training program was included (Kaats et al., 1998).

To give you an example of what happened to these subjects in an eight-week trial, one person lost only 1 pound on the scale; but she lost 9 pounds of fat and gained 8 pounds of lean mass and she also dropped a few dress sizes. Thus, improving her overall body composition. I've already described Juice Plus+®. Now, I'd like to tell you a little about the other two products used in this study.

- The **Juice Plus+ Complete®** protein/carbohydrate shake is a balanced blend of different sources of protein and low glycemic index carbohydrates. It doesn't have enough essential fats, as this would reduce its shelf life. Thus, I recommend that 1–2 tablespoons of omega-3-rich flaxseed oil (available in the refrigerated section of any health food store) be added per serving when making the shake. This mix can be blended with soy milk (for women[1]) (one with less than 10 grams of carbohydrate/more than 3 grams of fiber/more than 5 grams of protein per serving) or whole milk or plain water. Adding juices isn't recommended, because this would defeat the purpose of having a low glycemic index meal. A glass of juice has some 20 grams of carbohydrate, which acts like 60 grams because of the high glycemic index.

- **Juice Plus+ Thins®** is perhaps the most misunderstood product of the set. These are fiber wafers that contain natural ingredients that will help you to better regulate blood sugar. They will also help you to avoid another potential pitfall of the Atkins Diet®—depleting your glycogen stores. Remember, your brain and muscles depend on these glycogen stores. When you reduce your carbohydrate intake, you run the risk of depleting glycogen stores. These Thins® wafers have a fruit in them called "garcinia cambogia." This Asian fruit contains an ingredient known as hydroxycitric acid (HCA). HCA promotes the storage of glycogen by inhibiting the conversion of excess carbohydrates into stored fat in the body. Thus, using the Thins® is a great way to maximize glycogen stores and minimize the synthesis of —— body fat. When glycogen stores are full, the brain is happy

[1] Drinking soy milk is not advisable for men, young children or nursing mothers. Soy formulas are also not appropriate for infants.

and the craving for processed sugar goes down. Additionally, the fiber in the product will help to reduce the glycemic index of your meal. Both the long-term and short-term benefits of this product are phenomenal for helping the body reestablish hormone homeostasis. My only caution is to drink plenty of water. Remember, your body is being sculpted from the inside out. Be patient. Now that you are working *with* the body, and not against it, it won't be long until those jeans will fit again.

A review of the simple Longevity Eating Plan

When cave dwellers ate, they didn't eat much. It was real work to find food. What they found was fresh and raw. Since farming didn't exist, they had to keep moving for food and this not only provided exercise, but also, a variety of foods. Once the sun went down, they probably didn't have late evening meals and midnight snacks. There were no hydrogenated fat or food additives or colorings or flavor enhancers or preservatives or sugar added to their food. That was a simple eating plan. Our DNA had millions of years to adapt to this eating plan. Trying to change to a modern diet of processed foods is like trying to teach an old dog a new trick; our DNA doesn't understand. Remember the nomads in the movie *The Gods Must Be Crazy*? Even today, these African nomads are still eating a Stone Age diet. Now, you may not approve of their fashion sense, but you still have to admire their physiques.

Look, there's no way around it; you might as well start to love vegetables and make them the bulk of what you eat. Then, don't forget to have an adequate amount of protein (about the size of the palm of your hand) and your essential fats (1–2 tablespoons) *at each meal.* The usual choice should be whole foods, as Mother Nature made them. Start the day with a good breakfast, including protein, so that you maximize your metabolism and minimize the breakdown of lean mass. And don't eat too late at night. Remember to drink adequate amounts of pure, filtered water. It's not that hard to do. We're just creatures of habit; so, the only way to get rid of a bad habit is to replace it with a good habit. For example, if you focused all of your energy on trying to avoid drinking soda pop, you would keep having dreamy visions of a Coke®. Instead, you could get a gallon jug, fill it with filtered water, and play a game to see how long it would take for you to finish that jug. Similarly, empty your fridge and kitchen cabinets of junk food by filling them with whole foods. The bottom line is that food is not neutral. Our eating habits will either serve us or kill us.

13

Change of Heart

In the last chapter we discussed sarcopenia and how to avoid it through proper nutrition. In this chapter, we'll discuss how chronic stress can also contribute to sarcopenia. The end result of chronic stress and sarcopenia can be the onset of degenerative diseases such as heart disease, hypertension, depression, immune suppression, diabetes and degeneration of the brain. The Default Health Program leaves us exposed to the daily stresses of modern living, such as financial pressure, job security, time management, family dynamics and sitting in traffic. But each of us responds to those stresses differently. Some people have been conditioned by their early life experiences to handle stress better than others; but even those who might have had a less fortunate childhood can still reap the benefits of stress management by mimicking the behavior that comes naturally to these more relaxed individuals. The bottom line is that in order to achieve longevity, we need to "chill," to "take time to smell the roses," to "mellow out."

This is a lesson that was difficult for me to learn. In my

first year as a graduate student at Stanford, a new professor had joined the university—Dr. Robert Sapolsky. As first year students, we got to hear from each of the professors about the kind of research that he or she did, in order to make an informed choice about whom we would want as a thesis advisor. It was when Professor Sapolsky spoke to us about his research that I began to reevaluate my own propensity to get "stressed out." Somewhere along the way I had taken one of those self-scored personality surveys and had seemed to most closely fit the profile of a "Type A" personality. I had always considered this to be an asset, since it had allowed me to be a go-getter and to accomplish a lot. But then Professor Sapolsky talked to us about his ongoing studies of baboons in Kenya and what he was learning about the effects of psychological stress on their physiology. These baboons live in a national park and have no natural enemies. They get plenty of food. So any stress they experience is from social interactions. What I learned was that it was not easy to be an antisocial baboon in the Serengeti. If a baboon had friends, a good family life and had frequent grooming interactions, then life was good. Similarly, we humanoids tend to live longer if we have spouses or close friends—give or take the grooming (Sapolsky, 1999)[1].

Why would stress contribute to disease or a decrease in lifespan? It all has to do with something called the "fight or flight" response. Back in the good old days, if you had found yourself in the unfortunate position of meeting a lion for lunch at a local watering hole, this encounter would most certainly have induced this fight or flight response. Your adrenal glands would immediately have released

---

[1] Initially, I considered foregoing this chapter, since much of what I describe here is available in Sapolsky's book *Why Zebras Don't Get Ulcers*. However, I have chosen instead to give just enough examples to whet your interest, with the hope that you'll get a copy of this book for yourself.

steroids that would have mobilized your sugar and fat reserves—so that you could make a run for it! All this excitement would also have increased your blood pressure and heart rate. When you took off running, your body would have figured that you didn't need to digest your lunch, regenerate tissue and bone, or have sex during those few life-threatening minutes; so additional hormones would have impeded digestion, tissue and bone regeneration, and sexual response. Simultaneously, your brain would have begun to produce epinephrine to help your heart and other muscles work harder, and powerful opioids[2] to help you to suppress any sensation of pain. This remarkable chain of events in your body was designed to help you survive a dangerous situation. To this very day, as long as the perceived danger is short-lived, this fight or flight response contributes to our survival as a species. However, the opposite is true when we allow ourselves to feel stress all the time.

The fact is that the modern body responds the same way to an alarm clock jolting us out of bed in the morning or a threatening gesture from a fellow driver on the road as it would to being chased by a lion. Since chronic exposure to these stress hormones is harmful for the body over the long run, we need to control how we respond to modern stress in order to achieve longevity.

If we constantly challenge our digestion, this can lead to digestive disorders. For instance, say that you have two weeks to meet a deadline at work. The way your stomach chooses to help you out is to save some of the energy needed for proper digestion. The stomach cuts back on acid secre-

---

[2] Opiate drugs are exogenous analgesics, such as morphine and heroin. They bind to what are called opiate receptors that alter pain perception. The discovery of endogenous opioids such as endorphins, (which itself is a contraction of "endogenous morphines") occurred later, but the original opiate receptor name stuck.

tion and the proper maintenance of a strong a stomach wall. Then, let's say that once you've finally finished the work you had to do, you decide to relax and cook a nice meal at home. Now, under less pressure, your body is in a position to make more stomach acid again that evening; however, your stomach walls have thinned out during these past weeks leading up to the deadline and you find yourself experiencing acid rebound or acid reflux. Should this cycle of stress repeat a few times with the pressure of a few more deadlines to meet, then you'll be looking at an ulcer. This is just a brief example of how prolonged stress can play a factor in causing many types of digestive disorders.

Again, when the body discerns that we're stressed, it's going to look for ways to economize. But, it's not a good idea to shut down bone and tissue regeneration on an ongoing basis; the body needs to constantly rebuild itself, cell by cell, if it's going to stay healthy. The very stress hormones that are meant to ensure our survival can unwittingly induce bone loss and promote sarcopenia. Stress hormones redirect calcium from the bones, which need calcium for growth, to the kidneys for excretion. Additionally, stress hormones mess with the making of new bone cells and they slow down calcium uptake in the intestines from the food that we eat.

Stress hormones also contribute to sarcopenia by the way in which they affect insulin function. If you've been having trouble getting rid of your that beer belly or that tire around your waistline, you'd do well to look at your stress level for a clue. Mary F. Dallman of the University of California at San Francisco has studied how persistently high levels of stress hormones interact with insulin to increase food intake and to redistribute energy stores in the body. This results in more fat storage and less glycogen storage, neither of which is a good thing. According to Dallman, "the redistribution of energy stores from muscle to fat, particularly abdominal fat, may have a role in the development of abdominal obesity, which is strongly associated with increased incidence of adult-onset diabetes, coronary artery disease and stroke" (Dallman et al., 1995). Thus, stress hormones bias the body toward storing energy as fat instead of glycogen.

Prolonged stress also plays havoc with the immune system. Unfortunately, when the going gets tough—like losing a spouse, going through a divorce, or getting fired at work— we tend to get sick. Even minor life events can weaken the immune system. We can all cite examples from our own experience of catching a cold soon after taking a big exam or giving a presentation. Indeed, stress may make us more susceptible not only to the common cold (Cohen et al., 1997; Cohen et al., 1991), but also to the onset of autoimmune and inflammatory diseases and allergies (Elenkov and Chrousos, 1999).

In our society, it seems that working women, especially those with children, are more stressed than their male counterparts. In one study, both male and female professionals in high-ranking positions were observed for psychological and physiological stress responses related to work and family. Both sexes found their jobs to be stimulating and challenging; but the women seemed to have a higher stress response at work due to such factors as the "glass ceiling" when it comes to promotions or a greater workload for less pay. In addition, women with children had significantly higher stress hormone levels after work than the other participants, perhaps due to the fact that they never had a chance to unwind, even after they went home. Thus, these "super women" went to bed with elevated blood pressure and triglycerides as a result of their higher stress load. It seems that Type A women, myself included, need to consider the price we may be paying with our health (Lundberg and Frankenhaeuser, 1999).

One tricky aspect of stress is that your brain makes you numb to pain—a phenomenon called "stress-induced analgesia." Unfortunately, people get addicted to this euphoric state. I have experienced myself coming out of a stressful period, such as exam time, feeling worse than I did during the time I was stressed. This is a key component to understand. For example, one of my good friends had worked at a job for several years where she had not had enough time to eat proper meals. She had worked 14-hour days, sometimes 6 or 7 days a week, and that had left her with no time for a social life. Finally, she decided that a change was needed and found a job where she could make the same money by working 8-hour days only 3 days per week. Then, she found herself complaining about how her back was hurting and how she felt tired all of the time. She was perplexed by the fact that less work seemed to mean more pain. "What does it all mean?" she asked herself. Well, her brain had stopped making all those pain-suppressing opioids. I can imagine that about now you might be asking yourself, "Well then, what is the incentive to reduce stress in my life if it's going to be more painful?"

Excellent question; the answer is that the initial perception of being able to experience pain is a powerful signal from your body that damage has occurred while you were busily living a stressful life. Pain is, in fact, the only communication mechanism that the body has to alert the brain that something is wrong. *Numbing the pain by living a high-strung lifestyle or taking painkillers is akin to running red lights all the time, hoping that you'll never get into a collision.*

On the other hand, love is the antithesis of stress. Doing yoga, meditation, Tai Chi and spiritual practices may help reduce stress, but in the end I believe it's because they slow us down enough to sense the loving support that is all around us. I don't ever want to underestimate the value of the many paths that allow us to gain access to the experience of love.

When we find ways to increase the love we experience in our lives, we can undo, and even *prevent*, a lot of the premature aging process. "Of course," you say, "this is just good common sense," but this reasoning is also founded on sound research results.

- Animals that get a lot of attention during infancy handle stress better later in life.
- Adults with a rich social life handle stress better.

Scientists have a habit of being dry, using explanations such as:

The amount of maternal licking a rat receives during the first 10 days of life is highly correlated with the production of corticotropin-releasing hormone, the master hormone choreographing the stress response, in the hypothalamus of the brain of the adult offspring (Liu et al., 1997).

What they are really trying to say is that it's quite possible that if you had a mom who loved you and caressed you a lot during infancy, then you might be better programmed to deal with stress as an adult. Scientists also say stuff like, "The lowest levels of glucocorticoids are found in baboons with the strongest social networks" (Sapolsky, 1999). This really means that if you have a lot of friends who love you and/or a spouse who loves you and you love them back, then you are more likely to remain calmer during stressful times.

In the mountains of California, Doc Childre and his research team have been developing emotional self-management techniques that can be done in only a few minutes per day, and yet have been shown to alter a person's physiology for the better. They call it the HeartMath® system. According to the Institute of Heartmath®, these self-help techniques can reduce the harmful effects of stress hormones such as glucocorticoids; increase levels of helpful hormones such as DHEA; bring balance to the two branches of the body's nervous system, the sympathetic and the parasympathetic; and increase immune function.

All of this would seem to have obvious positive implications for one's health. So, what are these techniques? I have read several articles and have visited the Web site at http://heartmath.com to learn more about this program. The basic premise is that you can learn to:

- stop midstream during a stressful experience—Freeze Frame®
- check in with what is going on emotionally—Heart Lock-In®
- alter your existing emotional state by breathing, taking an emotional "temperature," and either recalling a loving (positive) past experience or imagining a heartwarming image—Cut-Thru®

These techniques are simple but effective. For instance, middle school children who participated in a course to learn these techniques demonstrated a continued ability to respond better to stressful situations, both outwardly in their behavior, as well as inwardly when physiological parameters were measured (McCraty et al., 1999). The heart, as it turns out, is not just the figurative seat of the emotion of love, but also the organ that can serve as the indicator of the stress response when we measure the variability of its pulse.

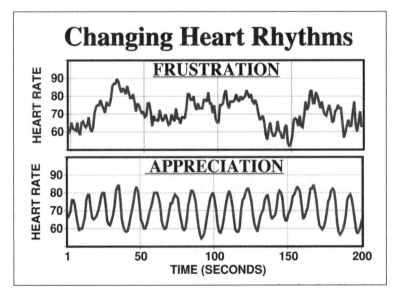

Figure 25. Changing heart rhythms by changing emotional state. Reprinted with permission. ©Institute of HeartMath Research Center.

The heart rate variability (HRV) is a measure of how errat-ic your heart beat is. For instance, when we say the heart is beating at 70 times per minute, in reality it may be beating at somewhere between 68 and 72 beats per minute; 70, then, is just the average. The heart rate variability is calcu-lated by measuring how much each beat varies from the average. The rate of the heartbeat is controlled by the nervous system. The *sympathetic* branch of the nervous system speeds up heart rate, as well as the adrenal glands (which secrete the stress hormones), respiration and other systems. The *parasympathetic* branch slows down the heart and other systems. Good health is a result of a balance between these two branches of the nervous system. During a stress response, the sympathetic branch becomes hyperactive rel-ative to the parasympathetic system and this state of imbal-ance can be directly observed by monitoring the heart rate variability. It is amazing to see how a quick exercise of managing the emotions can bring the heart rate variability back from an erratic pattern to a smoother, wavelike pattern.

I bring up Doc Childre's revolutionary research because of the implications of these simple, quick and inexpensive techniques. If you find yourself fretting in rush hour traffic, you could take two minutes to practice a little "Heart Lock-In®" and quickly change your mood. If you learned these tech-niques and practiced them every day, you could find your-self on the road to longevity. As they say at HeartMath®: "A change of heart changes everything."

When life starts to challenge you, whatever method you choose to slow down your breathing and manage your emo-tions of anger and frustration is great, as long as it works for you and you do it regularly. So remember, the next time you get mad at your spouse or workmate, think to yourself, "Is this really worth my getting so upset? Am I willing to risk catching a cold over this?" And not only do you risk a cold, but your increased levels of stress contribute to sarcopenia—the wasting away of your vital organs and lean body tissue—not to mention a host of other health problems, such as ulcers, heart disease, high blood pressure and diabetes. The incentive for learning to manage our emotional health is great—our very lives depend on it.

14

There was a crooked man...

I see a lot of people walking around crooked, suffering from chronic lower back pain and complaining about their chair or keyboard at work. Their wrists are also crooked, hurting from carpal tunnel and their eyes are going "crooked" from looking at the computer screen for too long. Then, there are women popping calcium pills as advised by their doctors, as a way of preventing the ultimate crooked state: osteoporosis. And when push comes to shove, diminishing budgets are forcing school authorities to cut back on gym classes for our children, while allowing soda machines and fast food franchises to come into the cafeteria—as a

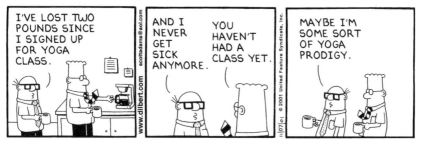

DILBERT reprinted by permission of United Feature Syndicate, Inc.

way to help out the schools finances. Crooked thinking. Can you ask for a better formula for fattening children, dulling their brains and giving them clogged arteries by age 10? Could it be that we aren't yet convinced about the benefits of exercise?

When I first started to write this chapter, I began with the premise that people already understood the benefits of exercise. I started to write the finer points of an exercise program for those who are already exercising. But, then reality hit me like a brick! But Mitra, what about the statistics of obesity, heart disease and diabetes? Are they an indication that most people are exercising already? So, I figured that like nutrition, there must be some myths about exercise as well, that need to be dispelled. And yes, I will eventually get to those finer points I mentioned; but let's start with some common myths that may be keeping you from moving your body (Report, 2000).

Myth #1: Weight gain is inevitable as you age. JoAnn Manson of Harvard Medical School says that weight gain with age is "a matter of reduced physical activity levels and lower metabolic rate caused by a loss of lean body mass." Researcher William Evans of the University of Arkansas agrees that "the lifelong loss of lean body mass reduces our basal metabolic rate as we age. It's very subtle change that begins between ages 20 and 30. The percentage of body fat gradually increases, and it produces an ever-decreasing calorie requirement." The end result is slow weight gain over decades. But it doesn't have to be this way. Exercise can mount a two-pronged attack on the expanding waistline. It increases the metabolism and, over time, it increases your lean mass. As your lean mass increases, your metabolism increases even more. Thus, persistent exercise can serve as a feed-forward cycle to help you achieve your ideal body composition at any age.

Myth #2: Strength training will make women too muscular. "Many women are afraid that strength training will make them bulky," says Miriam Nelson of the Jean Mayer U.S. Department of Agriculture Human Nutrition Research Center on Aging at Tufts University in Boston. Yet, women can benefit enormously from strength training without gaining enormous muscles. In one of Nelson's studies, postmenopausal women were randomly assigned to either do strength-training exercises twice a week or to do no additional exercise. After one year, the strength-training group had greater bone density, strength and lean mass, and a greater sense of balance. Women have less lean mass than men do and we've already discussed that lean mass includes your bones. This is why women are more likely to get osteoporosis than men. Nelson says that women need to take care of the lean mass that they have. "Thirty percent of middle-aged women have trouble doing physical tasks like walking a mile or carrying a few grocery bags or climbing a few flights of stairs. It's pretty staggering. They're really out of shape." But what about the big muscles? Women don't have the testosterone to make huge muscles. That's why many female bodybuilders end up taking steroids and testosterone supplements in order to compensate for not having the natural ability to build large muscles. This, of course, would *not* be a part of a regular strength-training program. There is now plenty of evidence supporting the fact that exercise is the strongest insurance against osteoporosis, while calcium supplements are a waste of your money.

Myth #3: If you can't exercise regularly, then don't bother. While it may take 10 weeks for you to increase your overall oxygen capacity, one day's worth of exercise can benefit your health. Give up your ideal of what regular exercise is. Start by exercising whenever you can squeeze it in. Stanford University researcher William Haskell says, "Take a 50-year-old man who is somewhat overweight and typically has moderately elevated blood sugar, triglycerides or blood pressure. A single bout of exercise of moderate intensity—like 30 to 40 minutes of brisk walking—will lower those numbers." These effects will last 12 hours or so. This may be why postal workers who carry mail have a lower risk of heart disease than postal clerks. Unfortunately, the picture-perfect exercise program that we create in the mind can sometimes keep us from that single, beneficial walk.

Myth #4: If you didn't exercise when you were young, then it might be dangerous to start when you're older, especially if you have a chronic condition. I'll remind you of the study I cited in *Chapter Twelve* done at Tufts University. Using frail nursing home patients, ranging in age from 87 to 96 years, this study showed that ten weeks of resistance exercise tripled muscle strength and increased muscle size by 10% (Evans and Rosenberg, 1992). Again Nelson says, "When they see what a difference it makes, they're thrilled." The same is true for people with chronic diseases. "People say they can't exercise because they have arthritis," Nelson adds, "but we see some of the greatest benefits in people with arthritis. Exercise reduces the pain and increases range of motion, strength and mobility." This doesn't mean that you should get off the couch for the first time and register for the next marathon in your area; it's important to start at your own pace and get professional help if you need some advice on what is your own pace. But it's even more important to *start*. Finally, for those of you who say that you don't have the time to exercise, I want to tell you that you're exactly right. Young or old, every sedentary day is reducing the time you have on this planet to be alive. So you can spend that time exercising or spend that time dead.

So, while there are really no good reasons not to exercise, there have been entire books written on the benefits of exercise. The next time you're tempted to say, "Oh, I don't have time. I'll just skip it today," I hope you'll remember this list of a dozen health challenges—backed by research—that can be alleviated by saying "yes" to exercise (Report, 2000).

1. **Sleep disorder**—A 16-week exercise program of 30–40 minutes of brisk walking or low-impact aerobics four times a week improved the quality, duration and ease of falling asleep in older adults who reported moderate sleep complaints but were otherwise healthy. Exercise reduces stress, relaxes the muscles and warms the body (King et al., 1997).

2. **Gallstones**—Active women are 30% less likely to have gallstone surgery than sedentary women. One study showed that women who spend more than 60 hours a week sitting at work or driving were twice as likely to have gallstone surgery as women who sat for less than 40 hours a week (Leitzmann et al., 1999).

3. **Colon cancer**—The risk of colon cancer is directly related to physical activity. Two studies show that sedentary people have twice the risk of active people (Giovannucci et al., 1995; Martinez et al., 1997).

4. **Diverticular disease**—One study showed that the most active men had a 37% lower risk of symptomatic diverticular disease than the least active men. Most of the protection against diverticular disease—the existence of pockets in the wall of the colon that can become inflamed—was due to vigorous activities like jogging and running, rather than moderate activities like walking; as an aside, the study also indicated that fiber in the diet was a key preventative factor (Aldoori et al., 1995). This is an example of how we have more reason to become more active with age, instead of less.

5. **Arthritis**—Regular moderate exercise, whether aerobic or strength training, can reduce joint swelling and pain in people with arthritis (Ettinger et al., 1997).

6. **Anxiety and depression**—Exercise releases powerful natural opiates that may help with anxiety and depression. One 10-week study showed that compared to a control group, moderate aerobic exercise four times a week improved people's aerobic fitness, and was associated with significantly greater reductions in tension-anxiety, depression and other moods than the control group; the subjects also reported being able to cope with stress better. These effects were maintained on a three-month follow-up visit (Steptoe et al., 1989). Another study examined the effects of exercise training on older patients with major depression. After 16 weeks, aerobic exercise was equally as effective as medication in reducing depression among patients (Blumenthal et al., 1999). All too

often, we resort to expensive medication when what the body really wants is a little movement. In my mind, depression and anxiety are usually good indicators of an inactive lifestyle.

7. **Heart disease**—Exercise prevents blood clots and promotes the breaking down of existing blood clots. Exercise also boosts the oxygen supply to the heart, creating tiny new blood vessels and expanding existing arteries. Many studies have shown that the risk of heart disease goes down with increasing fitness (Katzmarzyk et al., 2001; Manson et al., 1999). While even mild exercise is helpful, vigorous exercise can reduce risk of heart disease further (Ashton et al., 2000).

8. **Blood pressure**—A review of 22 studies shows that moderate exercise can lower or prevent high blood pressure. The average reduction in the better-designed studies was approximately 6–7 mmHg (millimeters of mercury) for both systolic and diastolic blood pressure, which makes exercise a comparable alternative to using pharmaceuticals to lower blood pressure (Arroll and Beaglehole, 1992).

9. **Diabetes**—In one study, women who walked at least three hours a week had about a 40% lower risk of diabetes than sedentary women. Once again, the more you move, the lower your risk (Hu et al., 1999).

10. **Falls and fractures**—Women 80 years or older, who were assigned to a strength and balance training program, had fewer falls and injuries than women who didn't exercise. Exercise has the potential to improve gait, balance, muscle and bone strength, as well as reaction time (Campbell et al., 1997).

11. **Enlarged prostate**—In one study men who walked

two to three hours a week had a 25% lower risk of enlarged prostate than men who seldom walked (Platz et al., 1998).

12. **Osteoporosis**—If you haven't gotten the message yet, exercise, especially strength training, increases lean mass, which includes bone density. A review of 62 studies showed that exercise-training programs prevented or reversed almost 1% of bone loss per year in both the spine and the neck for pre- and post-menopausal women (Wolff et al., 1999).

Now do you get it? No excuses. No weak bones about it. We need to get moving.

OK, now that I've convinced you about how important exercise is, I want to share with you some of the finer points that I've learned about exercise; these are perhaps not as widely known, and yet, are critical to any comprehensive discussion of longevity. I have spent my fair share of hours in the gym, grunting and sweating; but knowing what I know today, I'm convinced that I could have attained results more efficiently and without inflicting torture on my body. After all, "whipping yourself into shape" is only meant as a figure of speech. And yet, in the past, my fitness goals weren't attained without some harm done.

Whether you're an athlete already, a weekend warrior, or just getting started with exercise, I would like to bring the context of longevity to your exercise regimen. I'll be cheering you on to find the kind of exercise that really gets you excited, whether it's mountain biking, rock climbing, water aerobics or power walking. But, I'd hate to see you do your thing with a sore back and tight muscles. I'd also hate to see you start to look gaunt, to lose hair and to get sick all the time, just because you're trying to get in or stay in shape! I see too many athletes aging quickly, and I see no point in dying early on your way to getting fit. It's a fine balance, this fitness thing. By now, most of us have heard the phrase: "no pain, no gain." But in the rest of this chapter, we'll discuss how to work at your edge without jumping off the edge—in other words, we'll look at how to optimize your exercise program for maximum benefit without compromising longevity. Here are the topics we'll be covering.

- minimizing nutritional stress
- minimizing the release of stress hormones
- proper breathing and integrating mind and body
- warming up the body for exercise
- proper structural alignment
- increasing core strength
- finding your edge
- "sticktuitiveness"—if at first you don't succeed, try, try again

Minimizing nutritional stress

When I really committed to a fitness program, one of the first things that I had to learn was that frequent exercise didn't give me *carte blanche* to eat anything I wanted to eat. Yes, exercise does increase one's metabolism and need for calories; but most of us in America already eat too much anyway, and we do this without worrying about the quality of what we're eating. At all times, but especially when we embark on an exercise program, the food we select should meet the additional demands on the body. Before you allow any food to pass your lips, you should ask two questions:

- Will this help to combat the extra free radicals that my body is producing during exercise?
- Will this help my body to build more lean mass?

In the 1960s, exercise was not recommended for everyone, especially people over 40 years of age. But there was one man who spoke out vigorously to the contrary. That was Dr. Kenneth Cooper. With his book *Aerobics* he coined a new term for the form of exercise that he considered to be appropriate for people of all ages: "aerobic exercise." Aerobic exercise involves using oxygen to burn sugar for energy. You know you are exercising aerobically when your heart rate is up but you could still talk if you needed to. In contrast, you couldn't carry on a conversation during anaerobic exercise, such as quick repetitions of heavy weight lifting. This type of exercise leads to the build-up of lactic acid that makes for sore muscles the next day. Cooper had proposed that as far as aerobic exercise was concerned, "the more, the better" for everyone. In 1994 he qualified this philosophy in his book *Dr. Kenneth H. Cooper's Antioxidant Revolution*. After working with people at his famous Cooper Aerobics Center in Dallas, he realized that high-intensity exercise could promote more free radical production. But, according to Cooper, the solution is not to stop exercising, but rather to increase one's intake of antioxidants[1].

On the other hand, my attitude at the time was, "Hey, I was just slaving in the gym for an hour. Now I can go have ice cream." I'd like to reiterate here what we've already

---

[1] Cooper actually recommends a cocktail of antioxidants. But for reasons already stated in *Chapter 9*, I don't think it's necessary to take such a cocktail. Given the downside, I would recommend a whole food based supplement to augment the diet.

discussed about the value of micronutrient-rich macronutrients. I'm talking about the vegetables, fruits, lean protein, and good fats that are needed to support an active lifestyle. While exercise is fundamental to building lean mass and reducing body fat, it is proper nutrition that allows exercise to do its job. Here are some key things to keep in mind:

- You produce more free radicals when you exercise. This reinforces the need for a diet rich in vegetables and fruits and the whole food based nutrition available from the food concentrates found in Juice Plus+®.
- You need structural proteins and fats to build lean mass, and you need low glycemic index carbohydrates to supply consistent energy that will last not only during your workout, but throughout the rest of your busy day as well. Thus, avoid man-made carbohydrates and eat lots of fresh produce; make sure you eat sufficient amounts of a variety of proteins, as well as the good fats, as we discussed in *Chapter Eleven*. A Juice Plus+ Complete® shake made with 1–2 tablespoons of omega-3 flaxseed oil is a great pre-workout drink. I can't say enough about this shake as a way to increase the quality and length of your workout program. Most people run out of steam at around 20 minutes, when their glycogen stores run low. What can you do? Well, it's certainly not practical to stop for a big meal. So this low glycemic index/slow sugar-releasing pre-workout drink will make your workout more pleasurable. It's been clinically tested. It's helped Olympic athletes to win, and it can help you. In addition to the Complete® shake, there's another product called Juice Plus+ Thins® that can also help to regulate blood sugar. This program of whole food based

supplementation is an athlete's dream as far as "carbo-loading" and increasing lean mass to body fat ratio. It doesn't promise overnight results, but testimonials and research show that it sure works for those who stick with it.

- Finally, it's important to stay hydrated. The only thing that truly hydrates the body and powers its functions is pure water and the water found naturally in water-rich foods such as vegetables and fruits. I need to make an important distinction here: the latter is not an endorsement of vegetable and fruit juices. Juice alone, without the fiber, is a high glycemic index carbohydrate, which converts readily to sugar. And when sugar enters the body quickly, it dehydrates us[2]. This applies to fresh juice as well as pre-packaged juice.

Keep in mind that while proper nutrition can help you build a strong, lean body, improper nutrition can make you crooked: free radical damage to your joints and ligaments can lead to physical symptoms such as arthritis.

Minimizing the release of stress hormones

While strength training can be a great way to increase lean mass, too much weight or too many repetitions can make your body go into a fight or flight response, where you start to release stress hormones. Lift that dumbbell one too many times and your body will think that you are in real, physical danger—it will turn on that ancient survival mechanism. Up goes your blood pressure, pain tolerance, release of energy stores and down goes your immune system, DNA repair system, digestive system, and the chances of a good

---

[2] I do not endorse drinking juice regularly at all. I was glad to see a recent decision by the American Pediatric Society to take a stand for not giving children juice.

night's sleep. Again, balance is important: the right amount of exercise can help you sleep, while too much can keep you up at night. In the last chapter, we already discussed how this stress response causes long-term problems for your health. You certainly don't want your workout program to contribute to your daily stress load. Furthermore, if proper nutrition isn't there, this adds to the mess. Watch for these signs of overdoing it and not getting enough rest and nutrition:

- changes in your sleep patterns, especially insomnia
- longer healing period for minor cuts and scratches
- sudden drops in your blood pressure; dizziness when getting up from a seated position
- gastrointestinal disturbances, especially diarrhea
- gradual weight loss in the absence of dieting or increased physical activity
- a leaden or sluggish feeling in your legs during exercise
- impaired mental acuity and performance or an inability to concentrate
- the inability to complete routine exercise training sessions that were no special challenge previously
- an increase in your resting heart rate by more than 10 beats per minute early in the morning
- muscle and joint pains
- sluggishness that persists for more than 24 hours after workouts
- excessive thirst and fluid consumption at night

On the other hand, exercise routines that incorporate breathing and mindfulness with strength training, such as yoga and Tai Chi can actually reduce stress and stress-related risk factors for disease. For instance, exercise should increase your VO_2 max (which is defined as the maximum volume of oxygen consumed by the body each minute during exercise, while breathing air at sea level). Because oxygen consumption is linearly related to energy expenditure, when we measure oxygen consumption, we are indirectly measuring an individual's maximal capacity to do work aerobically.

In a study to compare the effects of Tai Chi on the circulatory system, elderly men (average age, 70) were instructed to practice an hour of Tai Chi for five days per week. Compared to a control group in their own community, these men who practiced Tai Chi increased their VO_2 max by 34%. Additionally, there were other improvements to their circulatory system, as in skin temperature, protective nitric oxide levels in their blood and blood flow (Wang et al., 2001).

And if you think you can't make time in your busy schedule for exercise because it's already too stressful, consider the following case study of 50 medical students preparing for final exams, certainly not a situation that lends itself to having plenty of free time to exercise. The students were instructed to practice yoga regularly and especially at times of increased stress. Participants showed a statistically significant reduction in anxiety levels and exam failures. Furthermore, student feedback surveys indicated that, compared to other students taking exams, the yoga group reported a better sense of well being, a feeling of relaxation; improved concentration, self confidence and efficiency; good interpersonal relationships; increased attentiveness; lowered irritability levels; and an optimistic outlook on life (Malathi and Damodaran, 1999). Do you think you might be able to make time for all of those benefits, after all?

Proper breathing and integrating mind and body

I was clueless about breathing when I first went to the gym. Yes, I tried to breathe during those "reps" of pushing and pulling weights and levers; but I never practiced and mastered breathing independent of anything else. That is, I didn't know and appreciate the importance of sitting still and doing nothing else but practicing my breathing, for its own sake.

The paradox is that getting faster results actually requires slowing down. I have nothing against joining a gym, but longevity does not necessarily look like that TV advertisement for a new health club that is opening in your town, with beautiful people pumping iron in beautiful clothes. Instead, longevity may be achieved by simply taking advantage of some ancient wisdom about exercise.

It's the single most important thing we do. And yet we hardly even think about it, unless we're running out. From our first to our last breath, life depends on breathing. The additional demands of exercise on the body require that we pay more attention to the way we breathe. The image of most western workouts involves a fast-paced breathing technique. Even elite athletes breathe this way during a race. But to breathe masterfully is to breathe slowly and steadily, filling the diaphragm from the bottom up, the way it was designed to work.

We are born knowing how to fill the entire diaphragm with air. But as we get older, we find ourselves taking shorter and shorter breaths, until the air barely makes it past the chest cavity; we tend to draw our stomach in and scrunch our shoulders up, collapsing the chest cavity inward. Rather than allowing the breath to enter, these movements deflate the diaphragm. During exercise, we continue to breathe in this constipated way, only at a slightly faster pace.

At the very time when we should be paying attention to our breathing, we are often trying to multi-task. We might read while on the stair-master or think about our daily challenges while running. Research has shown that paying attention while we exercise yields faster results than multi-tasking. Breathing is also the access to conscious exercising.

In yoga, consciously filling the diaphragm from the bottom up is called "Pranayama." *Prana* means energy and *yama* means discipline. Thus, Pranayama breathing is the discipline of bringing energy into the body. You may think that I'm starting to sound ethereal, but the oxygen we breathe in allows us to burn the food that we eat for energy. So, it would be good if we learned the discipline of bringing energy into the body. This ancient art form also says that the mind represents the future; the body, the past; and that the breath is the present. The practice of yoga, which means union, unites the mind and body through the breath, so that we can know the totality of our being in the present moment.

In the Default Health Program, the only sensation in our body that seems to demand our attention to the present is pain. To achieve longevity, we need to become more finely attuned to what is happening in each moment to our whole being—to be present. Since breathing purposefully makes us present, it is also the gateway to a deeper awareness of the structural alignment of the body and a quieting of the mind. I may sound like I'm digressing into spirituality—an area in which I wouldn't consider myself to be an expert—but yogic breathing also has very tangible healing properties. The power of yoga to heal or improve disease and illness is a new and emerging field of research. Already, preliminary studies are showing great promise.

In 1998, the *Journal of the American Medical Association* reported that yoga could improve carpal tunnel syndrome—a common complication of repetitive activity of the wrist. After eight weeks, yoga was found to be more effective than wrist splinting for relieving the symptoms (Garfinkel et al., 1998).

A year of yoga made a huge difference for a group of heart patients who had fewer anginal episodes per week, improved exercise capacity and better serum cholesterol profiles. Intervention with yoga was also shown to significantly reduce their need for coronary angioplasty or bypass (Manchanda et al., 2000).

Another study was designed to measure the influence of yoga on dexterity—quantified by the ability of a person to use tweezers to place metal pins in evenly spaced holes within a given period of time. This study showed that dexterity improved significantly in a group that began the practice of yoga, when compared to a non-practicing group

(Manjunath and Telles, 1999). Dexterity is a sign of a much more youthful brain. One of the most effective ways to maintain a sound mind and prevent neurodegenerative disorders such as Alzheimer's disease, is to keep the mind active and make it learn new tasks. The balancing poses of yoga provide this aspect, as well as increasing one's strength.

Another form of exercise that teaches proper breathing is the Pilates method of body conditioning created by Joseph H. Pilates. In Pilates (pronounced puh-LAH-teez) you learn to fill your diaphragm like a cylinder. You don't just fill it from the front. You fill it all around the body. Your ribs expand and your back muscles become relaxed and supple, allowing the breath to enter. Remember that learning to breathe properly takes practice. Voice lessons can also help to improve your breathing technique. Whatever the method or technique you select, invest at least 5 minutes before each workout session to focus on your breathing exercises. Then stay sensitized to your breath for the entire session. It is a lifeline for your body.

The importance of breathing became most apparent to me during labor. No form of physical activity that I have done has come close to how hard my uterine muscles had to work in order to deliver my babies into the world—not rock-climbing, not skiing all day, not going backpacking, nothing! I use this extreme example to show how powerful breathing can be. The uterus is comprised of different sets of muscles. These muscles work together to coordinate labor. There are vertically striped muscle fibers that form the outer layer; these are at the top and go over to the back of the uterus. These muscles contract to push the baby down. Then there are circular muscles fibers at the bottom, just above the opening; these work to open the outlet of the uterus and allow the baby to come out. The important thing is that these are big muscles that do a lot of coordinated hard work. Now, while the final stages of labor are usually very intense and pain is sometimes unavoidable, much of the pain experienced during the earlier process of labor can be avoided through slow and deliberate breathing. Such breathing provides an awareness of the body. Instead of grunting and moaning, this purposeful breathing allows a woman to actually visualize how these two sets of powerful muscles work together. This, in turn, allows her body to work more efficiently and conserves much-needed energy for the final stages of labor. Compared to resisting, grunting, huffing and puffing, slow and mindful breathing allows more oxygen to be available for the muscles to work aerobically. Acknowledging the pain and breathing through it is actually easier than resisting it—working against the body—and thereby experiencing more pain. What you resist will persist. When we fall short of oxygen, we are forced to depend on anaerobic metabolism and that can result in a painful build-up of lactic acid in our muscles.

So, what is a good basic breathing exercise? Well, you start by sitting comfortably and straight with your shoulders drawn back and your lower spine pulling down to the ground to straighten out your spine. You may want to sit against a wall at first until you become more accustomed to the process. Take a moment to focus on the way you're currently breathing. And then begin this guided breathing practice:

1. Completely exhale and let the stomach drop.
2. Then draw the breath in and expand the stomach naturally. You can put one hand on your stomach and one on your rib and continue inhaling till you feel your ribs expand.
3. Then exhale completely and let the stomach draw inward naturally.
4. Take another breath and this time move the hand that is on your stomach to your chest and continue to inhale until the breath fills your stomach, your rib cage and finally your chest cavity. Make sure your shoulders are not hunched up, but rather are rolled back and down, as well as relaxed.
5. When you exhale, let the air come out in the opposite direction, from your chest down to your stomach. Exhale completely until there is slight pause between your breaths.
6. Repeat this process for at least five minutes before each exercise session.

Breathing this way is not just important for exercise, but it is really how we should be breathing all the time. Eventually you'll breathe this way without even thinking about it, and the technique will not seem so exaggerated.

In contrast to holding the stomach in, breathing properly means allowing the stomach muscles to be at work, but in a relaxed and supple manner. I used to hold my gut in, thinking that this was the proper posture to hold and that it would make me look better in those slinky dresses. A sucked in stomach does not make for strong stomach muscles. Working your stomach muscles each and every breath helps to increase core strength. Also, stomach exercises should always be done with a conscious effort to keep those muscles supple and oxygenated, not tight and suffocated. Yoga instructors are known to remind us that a strong body is a relaxed body and a relaxed body is a strong body.

Warming up the body for exercise

Trying to work cold muscles is like trying to spread cold butter on toast; the toast breaks and the butter doesn't spread evenly. That is how we tweak a muscle and increase the chance of injury. I used to try to "stretch" a cold body, bent over, grunting and trying to reach my toes. Why? Because I was taught the importance of stretching before a workout. Then, I would wonder why my lower back would hurt later. In her book *Power Yoga*, Beryl Bender Birch explains that elite athletes get tight not from the intensity of the workout, but from not creating enough heat in their muscles during pre-workout stretching. As the wellness director of the New York Road Runners Club, she says that she has seen every kind of stretching program and exercise device and nothing has ever come close to being as complete, effective, thorough or well-rounded as astanga yoga. This ancient form of yoga dates back to somewhere between 400 and 200 B.C. (Birch, 1995).

The pre-workout warm-up session is a perfect time to practice your conscious breathing. One of my favorite forms of Pranayama breathing is called "Ujjayi" breathing. Beryl Birch believes that Ujjayi breathing actually helps to create heat in the body. To practice Ujjayi breathing, follow the sequence of breathing described earlier, except substitute the word "Khaa" as you breathe in and out. Then, close your lips gently, but maintain the same slight constriction of the throat as when saying "Khaa." Maintaining slow and even Ujjayi breathing during a workout creates heat and slows down the buildup of lactic acid. In fact, I used Ujjayi breathing during labor. Fortunately, there are now various types of slow and deliberate breathing techniques being taught in birthing classes.

Thank goodness that my normal workout program is a little easier than labor! As I said earlier, I cheer you on to pick the form of exercise that works best for you. But don't warm up with stretches. Like a stick of butter out of the fridge, your body isn't ready to spread out, and you'll eventually hurt yourself. Instead, start by standing still and focusing on your breath for 5 minutes. Then, do whatever exercise you were going to do, but modified at a slower pace. So, if you are going for a run, start with a brisk walk or a gentle jog. If you are going for a swim, swim at half the pace you normally can. If you are timing yourself, don't time the first 5–10 minutes of warm up. Starting more slowly will allow you the time you need to coordinate focusing on your breath with movement. Just like your car, you don't want to make a cold engine rev up from 0 to 60 mph without warming it up first. You also want a cool-down period at the end of each workout. Consciously cooling down will increase your ability to handle stress by bringing your stress hormones back into homeostasis. If you must stretch, stretch at the end, when the body is warmed up.

You may now be asking, "What about getting up to stretch when I've been sitting at my desk for a while?" Well, getting up and moving is a great idea, just *don't stretch cold muscles.* If you already know yoga, then I don't have to tell you about the benefits of breathing your way into a pose such as *Adho Muka Svanasana* or "downward facing dog." Even if you don't know yoga, practicing some simple breathing exercises would also help. I'd like to share another favorite Pranayama breathing technique that works especially well when you need to stretch at your desk or during long trips in a car or on an airplane. It's known as "Bhastrika"—the cleansing breath. It will also help to keep you awake if you're feeling tired.

1. Get comfortable in a chair or in your seat and loosen tight clothing or very tight seat belts.
2. Start by relaxing and breathing normally.
3. Now exhale forcefully and then begin to inhale deeply.
4. When the lungs are really full, exhale through your nose as quickly as you can. Assist this exhalation by contracting your stomach muscles. Using the stomach muscles is really important in this type of breathing.
5. Then quickly let the stomach relax completely as the air begins to come back in through your nose.
6. To fill the lungs again, exhale quickly through the nose, again with the aid of those stomach muscles. If the exhalation is really complete, you will find that the act of breathing in again is quite sudden and automatic, so that a rhythm is established.
7. Do this inhale-exhale pattern ten more times.
8. Depending on time constraints, you can repeat this cycle once more. As you get better with practice, you can work up to 90 breaths per cycle. That'll get things warmed up for you.

Proper structural alignment

Your new practice of conscious breathing will reward you with many benefits. When your breath has brought you more into the present moment, you may become more aware of how your body is responding to the demands of exercise. My first awareness of proper alignment came, as with breathing, from yoga. I had never realized how crooked my body really was until I got serious about my yoga practice. In the practice of yoga, the mind makes new connections as to how the body is supported through proper alignment. You'll be happy to know that proper alignment during any form of exercise can increase core strength and prevent injury. This new knowledge can also be applied in daily life; for instance, when you are sensitized to alignment, you might suddenly realize that you've been slumping at your desk. Knowing the value of proper alignment, you'll want to work on your posture. There are occupational therapists whose job it is to evaluate the effects of your work environment on your body, and to make recommendations for modifying your work habits. I've had physical therapists and chiropractors show me how to sit properly in a chair; but because it seemed like a lot of work, I never did it. Now through yoga, I've learned how to enjoy the freedom of having my body properly aligned. It is actually relaxing to sit properly. Once the body and mind become aware of the benefits of proper alignment, it's hard to go back to slumping in a chair.

Increasing Core Strength

Increasing your core strength is your doorway to a new level of fitness. Initially the goal of exercise is usually to get back in shape. Then we move to maintenance. But eventually, you may want to take it to the next level: you may aspire to become an elite athlete. In almost every sport, what sets the people at the top apart from the rest is that they have amazing core strength. So what is core strength?

I once heard a helpful analogy that compared core strength to the wheels on a car. Imagine a set of wheels that are made from the strongest materials in the world and are as polished and shiny in appearance as they are strong. In fact, the only thing wrong with these wheels is that their hubs are weak. The center hubs of these outwardly beautiful wheels are made out of plastic and beginning to crack. What's going to happen when we start driving a car on such wheels? No matter what grade of tires we put on these wheels, chances are, as the car goes faster, the hubs are going to break, the wheels are going to come off, and the car is going to crash.

An athlete's body is just like the wheel. No matter how strong the arms, chest, shoulders and legs look and feel, if the "core" (stomach and lower back) is weak, the athlete won't function properly. For explosive motions like jumping and sprinting, the upper and lower body must move in concert to generate maximum force. It is the muscles in the core that tie the upper and lower body together and help coordinate their motions. Athletes who possess a strong core will be able to better manage the motions of their bodies as they learn to perform at higher speeds. For instance, unless a runner works on developing core strength, he or she will eventually reach a plateau when it comes to speed.

You say you're not an elite athlete? For the rest of us, if you've ever wondered how to get better at your workouts—increasing your core strength is your access. As an example, my husband is a world-class athlete and I had resigned myself to the fact that no matter what sport we do together, I'll never catch up to him. When we go on hikes, I have to weigh him down with a heavy pack if I'm to have any hope of keeping up with him. Then I discovered the magic of increasing my core strength. I was attending a class in Hatha yoga at my local yoga studio, ostensibly to work on flexibility and relaxation, when I first got really focused on core strength and the difference it can make.

Pilates is another form of body conditioning that focuses on increasing core strength. So if this interests you, start doing your own research on who can train you to increase your core strength. Even on days when I don't have time for a full workout, I squeeze in 5 minutes of core work because the benefits are so great.

1. I lie down with my legs bent exactly 90 degrees at the knees and at the hips and practice breathing in and out, while constantly pushing my entire spine flat to the ground. This increases my awareness of the core muscles.
2. I raise both legs straight up, with my feet turned slightly out, but touching at the heel. I extend my body and especially my legs by imagining that I am reaching out through my heels and the crown of my head. The sensation is that of my hips and ribs separating, creating space in between them. Throughout this extension, I'm always aware of my breath and of relaxing my eyes, jaws, shoulders and neck.

3. I lower my legs slowly to the ground while exhaling. I keep projecting the balls of my feet and the crown of my head out from the center of my body until the exhalation is complete.

4. I inhale and raise my legs slowly back up to vertical, avoiding any tendency to swing them. If I become tired, it's better to raise and lower one leg at a time while keeping the other vertical, rather than to let go of my form.

5. I slowly and consciously repeat this 15–20 times, depending on how strong I feel—where my "edge" is.

The important thing with this workout is to engage the core muscles. I do some other variations by lowering my legs to either side of the body, sometimes with one leg crossed over the other. This is just to give you a taste of what core strengthening is all about. Should you try this at home, don't be disappointed if you can only do a few of them; this only means that you are following my directions really well.

For myself, I don't know if I'll ever be real competition for my husband who has always been an elite athlete and is over a foot taller than I am. But, at least now when we go for a hike, I am right on his heels instead of a mile behind him. Now I get to actually enjoy his company on those trails! Increasing core strength not only increases endurance but also increases fat metabolism and prevents lower back injuries. Strong core muscles help to hold structural alignment—that is, they help us run or walk a straight, instead of a crooked, mile.

Finding your edge

Every person has an edge—the place where you reap the most benefits without risking injury. How do you find it? Again, proper breathing and mindfulness are your access. For instance, have you ever tried to do a stretch and found it hard to do, until you took a deep breath, and suddenly something shifted and it got easier? What shifted was your edge. Your edge is different in the morning from what it is at night. Your edge is different today from what it was yesterday. Your edge differs from the left side of your body to the right. Your edge can change with every breath you take. The trick is to stay mindful during your entire work-out, find the place where an exercise seems just beyond your ability and then back off a bit. That's where it's safe but extremely effective to work out. For endurance athletes, finding the edge is an endless task. The edge will be different at the beginning of a race from what it might be in the middle, or at the end. Finding your edge is the same in this case as finding the right pace: fast enough to win but not so fast as to burn out. So even if you are just starting out, work at your edge. Don't bother trying to keep up with somebody else's edge. You'll become disappointed; or worse, you could hurt yourself. By focusing on your own edge, you will sense every time you move beyond it. To know your own edge is a very empowering thing.

If at first you don't succeed, try, try again.

I'd like to end this chapter with what, I believe, is the most important component of any successful exercise program: commitment. A commitment to exercise, as it turns out, does not happen overnight for most people.

Sometimes it means recommitting, over and over again. The good news is that those who have had success have found it to be a series of stops and starts. Psychologists and fitness experts have found this pattern to be a nearly universal process that starts with ignoring or discounting exercise, to an on-again, off-again pattern, and finally regular exercise (Fenton and Feury, 2000). So wherever you are in this journey is the perfect place to continue moving forward towards longevity.

Conclusion: From Here to Longevity

These are exciting times. More and more healthcare professionals are making a shift towards prevention. The leading science journal *Nature* published an article by renowned cell physiologist Dr. Leonard Hayflick entitled "The Future of Ageing." In this article Hayflick writes that research on age-related diseases has outpaced our understanding of the fundamental disease process (Hayflick, 2000). According to Hayflick, "Determination of longevity must be distinguished from ageing to take us from the common question of why we age to a more revealing question that is rarely posed: why do we live as long as we do?" In other words, we would do best to study the healthy body, how it works and how to keep it healthy. We should study living rather than dying.

In this book, I've made a case for why it would probably serve us better to focus on how to keep the healthy cells healthy, as opposed to worrying about the symptoms caused by the cells that are sick. In order to break from the Default Health Program, I suggest that we need to forge a new alliance.

We, as individuals, agree to accept responsibility for our own health, leaving researchers and clinicians more time to focus on longevity.

In *Chapter Two*, I described a new way to look at disease. Disease is often caused by environmental and lifestyle factors that tamper with proper DNA expression and proper enzymatic function. The important concept is that modern medicine looks at health from the wrong end, the diseased leaves and branches of the Default Health Program Tree. The number of field specializations in medicine and medical technology continues to increase, with a concurrent rise in the number of people who are suffering from age-related diseases. It just doesn't make sense to continue to focus so much of our research on the diseased branches, and then wonder why there is no fruit. You don't need a green thumb to understand that we should be looking at what is feeding the root system. Only trees that have received plenty of pure water, adequate nutrients, sunshine and clean air can hope to bear the fruit that Nature intended. Why should we be any different?

For instance, I saw a public television special on emotions and the brain. An overview of the show read:

Emotion is now considered integral to our over-all [sic] mental health. In mapping our emotions, scientists have found that our emotional brain overlays our thinking brain: The two exist forever intertwined. There is a critical interplay between reason and emotion. We are well aware of how brain malfunctions can cause pain, depression, and emotional paralysis. We must also understand that the brain affects positive emotional responses such as laughter, excitement, happiness, and love. Scientists have been able to pinpoint the section of the brain that causes laughter (with no intention of finding a cure!) (PBS series, 2002).

Ironically, the show only featured people with depression and post-traumatic emotional disorders. The overview had given me the impression that I would have a glimpse into the study of emotions from a positive angle. Upon actually viewing the show, I was disappointed to find that no mention was made of any studies on why people *don't* suffer from depression or why some people become emotionally paralyzed after a life-threatening experience while others do not. For example, I think it would be enlightening to inquire about the antioxidant status, hormone profile, diet, sleep patterns and exercise patterns of people who get into major traffic accidents. We might see a trend in what factors are important to prevent post-traumatic emotional disorders. That is, maybe eating your veggies doesn't just protect you from age-related diseases, but perhaps it might also prepare you to withstand physiological and psychological trauma better. As discussed in *Chapter Seven*, if a fetus survives stress better with proper nutrition, why wouldn't we continue to benefit from nutrition outside the womb?

In one segment of the show, a woman was interviewed whom psychiatrists consider to have an incredible success story with antidepressant drug treatment. While she conveyed her anxiety about her dependence on the drug and her need to increase the dosage eight-fold over a twelve-year period, she also credited the drug treatment with allowing her to function in society. She reported that after treatment, she went from being a lonesome regular at her local hospital, to getting married, having a child, getting a professional degree in psychology, practicing psychology and writing a best-selling book. That's quite a testament to the potential power of antidepressants. My only question is why was there no discussion on the show of any consideration of her need to exercise, eat right and rest—all of which would naturally increase the production of desirable "emotion hormones" such as serotonin and epinephrine. What if she had been encouraged to make the lifestyle changes that could have kept her from needing to increase the dosage of the antidepressant? What if she had known how much power she has over her own recovery?

In the course of this book, we've talked about current cancer research aimed at identifying more of the genes that are linked to cancer. I'd like to suggest that researchers will probably never have a definitive list. If we continue, as a society, to add insult to the injury that our genetic material has already sustained, even more of the mutations that cause cancer are bound to occur. The bottom line is that there may be an infinite number of pathologies and disease states that we can expect to develop from the large number of DNA mutations that can occur. For example, we discussed the importance of proper gene expression. Sometimes proper expression means *no* expression; that is, it can be equally important to silence the expression of certain genes for the body to function properly. A case in point would be genes that cause cells to continually grow and divide; the over-expression of such genes might lead to cancer.

One of the ways that the body accomplishes this silencing is through a process called methylation of the DNA. The nutrient folic acid is critically important to the proper methylation of DNA, such that even a slight deficiency can cause hypomethylation. "Hypo" means less than normal; that is, the silencing process will be retarded. This can have widespread consequences as any and every cell in the body might be erroneously expressing DNA that shouldn't be expressed, resulting in any and every kind of disease. Indeed, specialists from all of the major fields of medicine— psychiatry, oncology, neurology, gerontology and cardiology —all have published hundreds of papers on the effects of folate deficiency (folate is the same as folic acid) and the complications resulting from hypomethylation. And in every case it took time and money to trace the disease state back to that folate deficiency. You can get more folic acid by eating more produce. But if you don't always get your 5–9 servings of vegetables and fruits every day, you'll be glad to know that taking Juice Plus+® is another excellent way to help you get the folic acid your body needs.

As I mentioned, there are numerous disease states that have been traced to a folate deficiency. For our purposes, let's begin by looking at cancer, and cancer research specifically. There are many cancers to be studied. There are therefore many researchers, each tending to specialize in a particular type of cancer. Within each of these specializations there are those who approach a certain type of cancer, say breast cancer, from a molecular or cellular perspective; others who study the epidemiology of breast cancer; and still others who study the clinical aspects of the disease. Now, this happens for every type of cancer. Meanwhile, there is a simple, common theme emerging from the preventative point of view: folate deficiency can increase the risk of all cancers (Choi and Mason, 2000).

It is easier for us to take steps to avoid folate deficiency than to look at the disease state and try to trace it back to what went wrong. It seems so arbitrary to study health from the perspective of disease. While such research often provides information about how a disease occurs, we still have no cures for heart disease, stroke, cancer, diabetes, and the many other ills that plague us.

Preventative research is currently not "sexy" research. By that I mean that we, as a society, are mostly still looking for miracle cures. Most people are still hoping that someone else will ultimately take responsibility for their health. For those of us who are willing to step up to the plate, there is good news. And I'm assuming that this includes you, since you've taken the time to read through this book. If you decide today to start treating your body like a temple, chances are that it's not too late. An article in *Time* magazine gives what I think are some very hopeful examples of just how quickly the body responds to positive changes in lifestyle (Gorman, 2001).

- Lab measurements show that increasing your intake of fruits, vegetables and fiber changes the blood's sensitivity to insulin within two weeks, reducing the risk of diabetes almost immediately.
- Scientists find that sedentary 40-year-old women can reduce their risk of heart attacks to almost the same level as women who have exercised conscientiously their whole

lives by starting a program of walking briskly for one half hour a day, four days a week.

- If you smoke, on the day that you decide to quit, you will reduce your carbon monoxide levels dramatically. A week later your blood will become less sticky, making it far less likely that you will suddenly die of a heart attack. While the risk of heart disease still exists for past-smokers, four to five years of abstinence will reduce the risk of a *fatal* heart attack to as low as someone who has never smoked.
- Women who consume as little as 8 oz. of fish a week can cut their risk of a stroke by half.

The article also points out that we have our work cut out for us in terms of taking personal responsibility. Fifty million Americans still smoke. More than 60% of Americans are obese or overweight; 25% get no exercise at all. At best, 25% eat the recommended minimum of five servings a day of vegetables and fruits; although I've read other sources that say that it's less than 9% who do eat enough produce. The incidence of diabetes is on the rise. In light of this less promising information, I'd like to reiterate that achieving health and vitality is a journey; just as we may have to recommit again and again to an exercise program, the rest of our health program may also have many starts and stops before it gains momentum.

We're only just beginning to appreciate some of the advantages of living a simpler life—more like that of our Stone Age predecessors. For instance, another way that our body silences genes is through the acetylation of an area of our chromosomes called chromatin. It turns out that we need a chemical called butyrate to achieve proper acetylation of chromatin. Now butyrate is a fatty acid that is produced by the fermentation of friendly bacteria that live in insoluble fiber in our gut. So anything that inhibits the growth of this bacterium can affect the proper expression of DNA in every cell of the body and thereby cause a multitude of diseases. If you don't get enough fiber in your diet or if you take antibiotics too often, your body becomes a playground for DNA foul play. Okay, so you could have gone all day without thinking about what is going on in your gut. I know this is not sexy, high-tech biotech, but it elucidates how much control we have over our own health. Eaten any good fiber lately?

Another bit of good news is that a few brave researchers and clinicians are looking to help us out from the preventative point of view. There are more and more nutraceuticals emerging on the market. In contrast to pharmaceuticals, nutraceuticals provide therapies that are being developed for specific ailments and can enhance the body's own ability to repair the damage. After all, the body already has a very sophisticated mechanism in place to repair DNA, and as long as environmental and lifestyle insults do not overburden this mechanism, most of us should be able to lead a long and productive life. You can't imagine the screening your DNA was subjected to in the process of going from sperm and egg to a viable fetus. The point being that you have much more that's working in your body than is not working; and the fact that you're here and alive is the living proof.

We need to be doing everything that we can do, every single day, to protect the healthy DNA that we have. We've already talked about the power of vegetables and fruits to do this. This power has been concentrated in whole food based products like Juice Plus+®, which consistently gives the body the micronutrients from vegetables, fruits and grains everyday. Preliminary research suggests that supplementation with this product goes a long way towards protecting the DNA of our cells. Just think, before whole food based products, all we had were vitamins. One doctor took it upon herself to study her patients who were suffering from degenerative diseases and already taking supplements, in order to see if their health improved after adding Juice Plus+® to their daily regimen. She published her results, showing that whether patients had taken inexpensive vitamins or expensive, tailor-made antioxidant supplements, adding Juice Plus+® improved their overall antioxidant protection level by 240% (Ellithorpe, 2001).

In addition to the Juice Plus+® products, I would advise anyone to also take some essential fatty acid supplements. Many companies market excellent essential oil products. This supplement combination should provide any diet with what I consider to be the three missing links as far as nutrition is concerned—whole food phytonutrients, essential fats and complete protein.

In the very first chapter of this book, I posed many of the questions that we all seem to have about our health. I hope to have answered some of the most fundamental ones. Still, other questions may remain, such as questions about immunizing children. This discussion would require another book—so shortly I'll recommend one to you. First, I'll add my two cents worth. Immunizations have been one of medicine's victories. Today, children suffering from polio, mumps, measles, diphtheria and whopping cough are rare compared to the middle of the twentieth century. The difference between an immunized child and a non-immunized child is clear when we compare the number of protective antibodies found in the blood of a child after he or she has been weaned from mother's milk. The immunized child is better protected than the non-immunized child from the standpoint of a well-primed immune system as a result of the immunization (Zinkernagel, 2001).

But, does this mean that parents should blindly follow the recommended schedule for immunizations—some 33 doses of 10 vaccinations in the first five years. Such a planned invasion should raise questions for any concerned parent. For any parent struggling with the pros and cons of vaccinating a child, I recommend an excellent book that has gathered the most up-to-date information that is available regarding immunization. *What Your Doctor May Not Tell You About Children's Vaccinations* by Stephanie Cave, M.D. (Warner Books, 2001) explores a parent's options, such as alternative immunization schedules and toxin-free immunizations. If, after reviewing all of the information, a parent should choose against vaccination, the book also supports that decision by guiding the parent through the often complicated process of seeking medical waivers and exemptions. According to Dr. Cave, vaccines are a big business—over $7 billion dollars worth in 2001; so it's worth finding out what kind of real protection we are buying for our children.

Because of advances such as childhood immunizations,

the average person is living longer; unfortunately, we are also experiencing the health consequences of a lifetime of lifestyle choices and environmental hazards. Quantity of life is not enough. Many of us are wondering what we can do to ensure that we also enjoy a *quality* of life. Recently, I had the pleasure of hearing one of the most recognized and frequently cited scientists in the world—Dr. Bruce Ames (I've already cited him often in this book). He spoke on the topic of micronutrient deficiencies in our diet (Ames, 2001). While Ames made a strong point that we should eat our vegetables and fruits, he also suggested that there are currently supplements that can reduce the effects of aging in every cell of the body. He discussed the process whereby the body produces energy to support its many functions. The mitochondria, which are the energy-producing batteries inside our cells, burn metabolites; and the natural consequence of that is the production of toxins, known as free radicals. According to Ames, compounds such as R-Lipoic Acid and acetyl-L-carnitine have been shown to reverse the damage done by free radicals. If they can help make old laboratory rats get up and do the Macarena, then perhaps eventually we humans can also extend our active and productive years[2]. *What intrigues me about this research is that it is aimed at improving the state of every cell in the body; this research exemplifies the hybrid philosophy that it is possible to have a molecular understanding of a holistic approach.* Mechanism meets Vitalism and they shake hands in this approach to research.

Going back to Hayflick's article on "The Future of Ageing," he considers what will happen if we do suddenly

---

[2] Acetyl-L-carnitine and the R isomer of Lipoic Acid, separately enhance youthful markers in rats. They both reduce levels of oxygen radicals and aldehydes from lipid peroxidation. They both increase levels of cellular ascorbate and glutathione. When given together, the "anti-aging" effects are larger in general.

find "a pill" to stop aging. After all, we have increased the average lifespan or life expectancy. The consequence of increasing average lifespan has been that there are more people living to the point of frailty and dependence. So Hayflick considers whether it would be wise to unlock the mysteries of mortality if it means using more resources to take care of more old people. He cautions, "Biogerontologists have an obligation to emphasize that the goal of research on ageing is not to increase human longevity regardless of the consequences, but to increase active longevity free from disability and functional dependence."

I believe that the latter will happen automatically. Why? We already have a balance of lifestyle-inflicted damage vs. anti-aging mechanisms in our body. Even if there were such a thing as a longevity pill that could reduce the damage of aging, all that a pill could hope to do would be to reset the balance point of damage vs. repair. Longevity and the freedom from disability and dependence must go hand in hand. I don't think it's possible for the majority of the population to enjoy living beyond a hundred years unless we first retard the damage that is being done to our DNA, and thereby slow the advance of degenerative disease. Genetic disposition or the magic pill will not be enough to maximize our full potential. We have to get involved in directing our own play.

And we *can* direct our own play. For example, if we look back to *Figure 8* in *Chapter Eight*, we see that, other than "Genetic factors" and "Normal metabolism," all of the other factors that can tip the balance of our antioxidant status are in our control. Thus, I present to you the Longevity Tree. This figure points us to the ways in which we can feed the very roots of health. For instance, our Stone Age ancestors didn't have to be wise about the foods they ate, other than to avoid poisonous foods such as toxic berries and plants. These were generally bitter and as such, easy to distinguish. Sometimes, their food might have been contaminated with invisible deadly microbes—unless a food is rotting, it's hard to distinguish when lethal microbes might be present. Other than these considerations, what they ate served the body well: freshly hunted meat or fish and freshly picked plant life. From an evolutionary perspective, we are "unarmed"

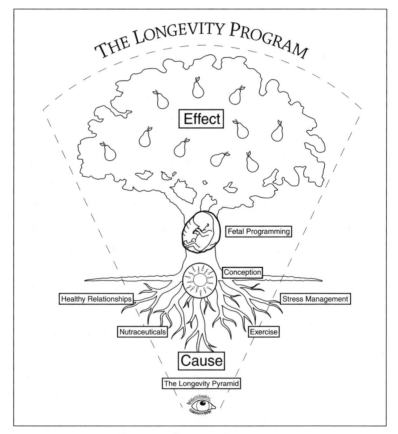

Figure 26. The Longevity Program

when we see "fast food" or processed food. We have not adapted to the modern toxic food environment. For instance, it's inconceivable to our genes that something that tastes sweet, like ice cream or a cookie, could be harmful to us. *We have no pre-programmed relationship to modern, toxic foods.* It is only those who seek out the information who learn to eat discriminatingly.

Today, the "rich fat man" is an oxymoron. Studies show that those who enjoy financial success also enjoy health. They have the luxury to become health-conscious—aware of their own health and the factors that contribute to their state of health. But those among us who are so fortunate should consider that until *all people* enjoy the simple basic needs of life—security and health for themselves and their families—there will continue to be dangerous conflict in the world, from which no one is ultimately safe. Thus, I urge each and every one of you to take a stand, not only for your own health, but also for the health of all people everywhere.

So, get to it!

Suggested Reading

Chapter 2

Fast Food Nation: The Dark Side of the All-American Meal by Eric Schlosser (Houghton Mifflin, 2001). For author/reporter Schlosser, what began as an article for *Rolling Stone* on the fast food franchise industry soon became a book. If you are brave enough to deal with the real scoop on the fast food establishments, this is a must read.

Chapter 3

Over Dose: The Case Against the Drug Companies by Jay S. Cohen, M.D. (Tarcher/Putnam, 2001). Dr. Cohen is an associate professor of family and preventative medicine at the University of California, San Diego. In this book he explores "the poor research methods on the part of the drug companies" and "the deliberate effort to create easy, one-size-fits-all dosages that both appeal to doctors and produce inflated effectiveness statistics."

The Crazy Makers by Carol Simontacchi (Tarcher/Putnam, 2000). This book explores the role of food in childhood development, particularly as it affects the brain.

Chapter 5

The website—http://www.rco.on.ca/factsheet/3Rhome.html— offers these helpful fact sheets:
- Household Hazardous Waste
- How to Have a Greener and Cleaner Spring
- Recycling Activities for Children
- Home Made Paper Recipe
- Indoor Plants as Air Purifiers
- Safer Alternatives for Toxic Products
- Ideas for Organic Lawn Care and Gardening
- Make Every Day Earth Day
- Facts & Stats on Cars

Chapter 8

Antioxidant Status, Diet, Nutrition and Health by Andreas M. Papas (CRC Press, 1999). I recommend this for the technically minded. It is a dense, but informative book and is well worth the read.

The Antioxidant Revolution by Kenneth Cooper, M. D. (Thomas Nelson Publishers, 1994). Explores the relationship of exercise to antioxidants, offering insight into why exercise is not beneficial unless the diet matches the workout.

Why Zebras Don't Get Ulcers by Robert M. Sapolsky (Freeman, 1999). While somewhat technical, a well-researched and well-documented book written with a lot of wit.

Chapter 11

"The Myths of Vegetarianism" by Stephen Byrnes published in the July 2000 issue of the *Townsend Letter for Doctors and Patients*. You can usually access this article on the Web by doing a search for the author's name and the term "vegetarianism." This is an excellent and comprehensive article that not only discusses the nutritional concerns, but also covers the socio-political and environmental issues around vegetarianism.

Eat, Drink and Be Healthy by Walter C. Willett, M.D. (Simon & Schuster Source, 2001). This comprehensive book tells you why the USDA Food Guide Pyramid is wrong. As it says on the cover: "Not merely wrong, but wildly wrong. And not just wildly wrong, but even dangerous." Dr. Willett's conclusions are based on decades of research by Harvard Medical School and Harvard's School of Public Health. Full of informative charts and graphs, it's a good resource to have in your library.

Chapter 12

Beating Overeating: The Lazy Person's Guide by Gillian Riley (Newleaf, 2001). This short and sweet book shows you how to strengthen your motivation, and how to handle the feeling of being deprived and tempted by all that food you don't really need.

Quitting Smoking: The Lazy Person's Guide by Gillian Riley (Newleaf, 2001). Another great, short book explains a very straightforward technique to think yourself through the process of quitting, paying particular attention to how to stay "stopped" long term.

Sugar Blues by William F. Dufty (Warner Books, 1976). This timeless book is a dose of reality on how addicted we are to sugar. It warns us about the addictive quality of sugar.

Chapter 14

Here are two great books on breathing:

Breathing Your Way to a Revitalized Body, Mind and Spirit by Guruchara Singh Khalsa (Broadway Books, 2001).

The Tao of Natural Breathing: For Health, Well-Being and Inner Growth by Dennis Lewis (Mountain Wind Publishing, 1997).

Conclusion

What Your Doctor May Not Tell You About Children's Vaccinations by Stephanie Cave, M.D. (Warner Books, 2001). Dr. Cave, an expert on pediatric vaccinations, is concerned that we may be overvaccinating our children today. The book cover reads: "Once considered a godsend, vaccines are now felt by some to be associated with dramatic increases in brain and autoimmune diseases such as autism, asthma, diabetes, learning disabilities and ADHD." This is a vital, down-to-earth guide that will tell you which vaccines may be risky and what you need to consider in order to safely vaccinate your children.

Figure Reproductions

Several figures used elsewhere in the text are reproduced
here in color. In some cases, they have also been enlarged
and/or enhanced or positioned for easier comparison.

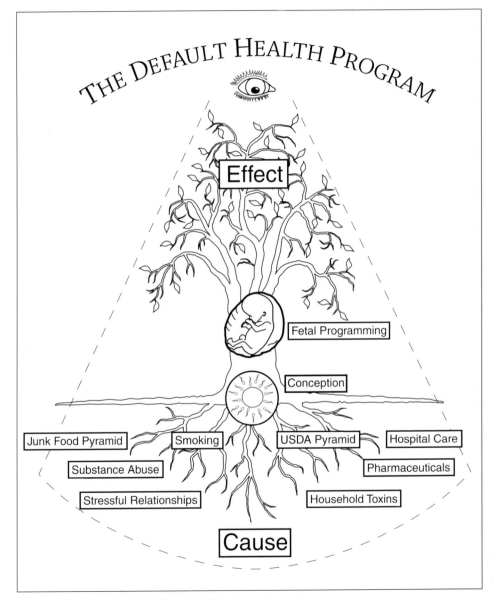

Figure 1. The Default Health Program

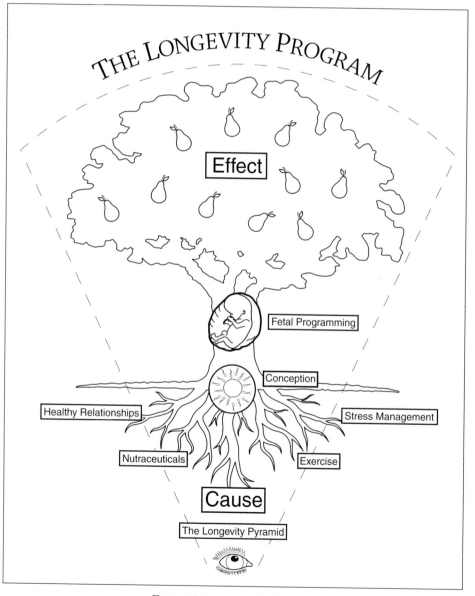

Figure 26. The Longevity Program

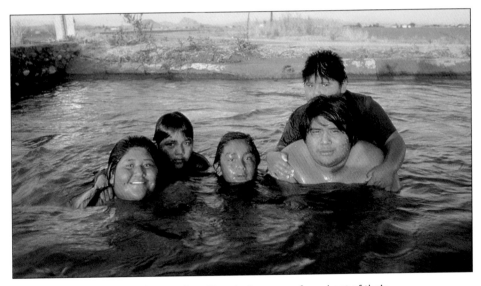

Figure 4a. The American Pima Indians were forced out of their traditional lifestyle in the 1970s and now have the highest incidence of obesity in the world.
Reprinted with permision from John Annerino. Copyright ©2001.

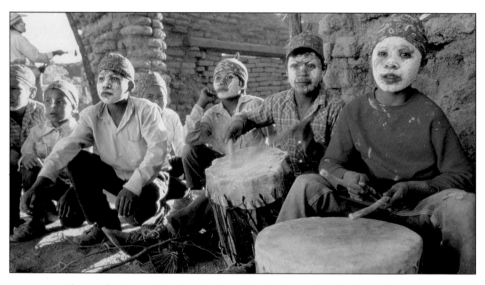

Figure 4b. Meanwhile, the Mexican Pima Indians, who also have the same "thrifty genes" that like to store fat, are on average 57 pounds lighter as a result of being able to continue with their original active lifestyle and a diet more suited to their genes.
Reprinted with permision from John Annerino. Copyright ©2001.

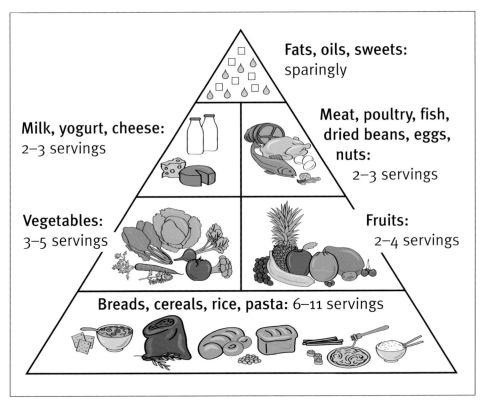

Figure 13. USDA Food Guide Pyramid

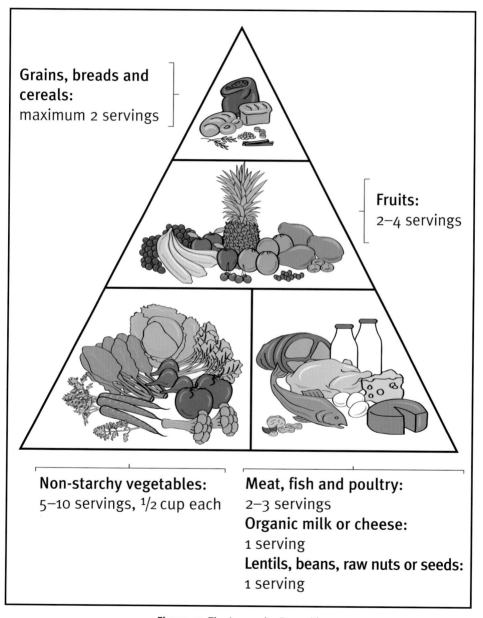

Figure 21. The Longevity Pyramid

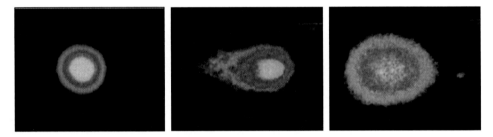

Figure 6. Typical undamaged control nuclear DNA (left); moderately damaged nuclear DNA (middle); and heavily damaged nuclear DNA (right). Images are oriented with nucleus to the right and migration of DNA to the left. Reprinted with permission from Elsevier Science; see *Selected Bibliography* (Smith et al., 1999)

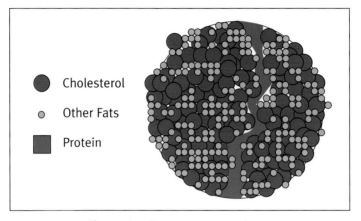

Figure 16. Schematic Diagram of LDL

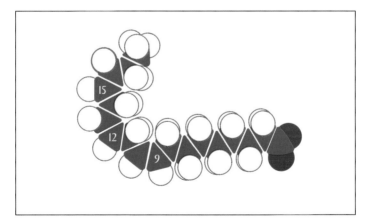

Figure 18. Space-filling model of linoliate, a poly-unsaturated fatty acid with three cis double bonds; the carbon atoms are in blue, hydrogen in white and oxygen in red. There are cis double bonds between carbons 9 and 10, between 12 and 13, and between 15 and 16.
Reprinted with permission of W.H. Freeman and Company from BIOCHEMISTRY by Lubert Stryer. ©1988 by Lubert Stryer.

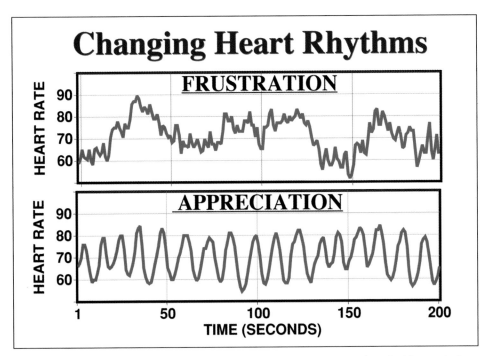

Figure 25. Changing heart rhythms by changing emotional state. Reproduced with permission. ©Institute of HeartMath Research Center.

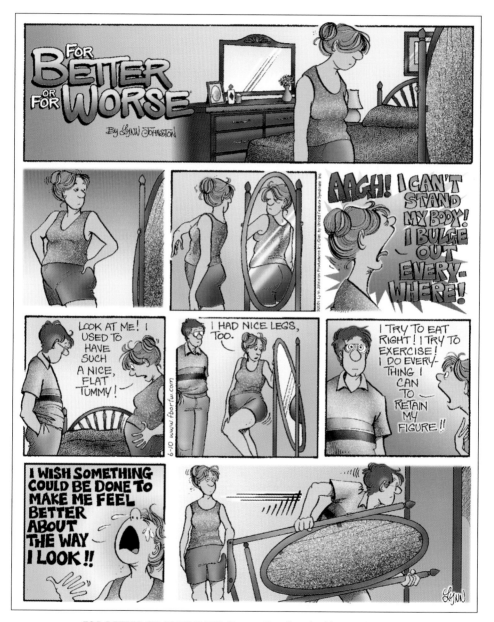

FOR BETTER OR FOR WORSE ©2001. Reprinted with permission of
Lynn Johnston Productions, Inc. All rights reserved.

Selected Bibliography

Chapter 1

Davenas, E., Beauvais, F., Amara, J., Oberbaum, M., Robinzon, B., Miadonna, A., Tedeschi, A., Pomeranz, B., Fortner, P., Belon, P., et al. "Human basophil degranulation triggered by very dilute antiserum against IgE." *Nature* 333, no. 6176 (1988): 816–18.

Maddox, J., Randi, J., and Stewart, W. " 'High-dilution' experiments a delusion." *Nature* 334, no. 6180 (1988): 287–91.

Torti FM, Adams KM, Edwards LJ, Lindell KC, Zeisel SH. "Survey of Nutrition Education in U.S. Medical Schools—An Instructor-based Analysis." *Med Educ Online* [serial online] 6, no. 8 (2001). Accessed 2002. Available from: http://www.med-ed online.org/res00023.html

Wells, H. *Homeopathy for Children*. Boston, MA: Element Books, Inc., 1993.

Chapter 2

Anderson, R. N. *US Decennial Life Tables for 1989–91*. Hyattsville, MD: National Center for Health Statistics, 1999.

Hayflick, L. "The future of ageing." *Nature* 408, no. 6809 (2000): 267–9.

Kirkwood, T., and Austad, S. "Why do we age?" *Nature* 408, no. 6809 (2000): 233–8.

Puca, A., Daly, M., Brewster, S., Matise, T., Barrett, J., Shea-Drinkwater, M., Kang, S., Joyce, E., Nicoli, J., Benson, E. , et al. "A genome-wide scan for linkage to human exceptional longevity identifies a locus on chromosome 4." *Proc Natl Acad Sci U S A* 98, no. 18 (2001): 10505–8.

Chapter 3

Avila, J. "High cost of prescription drugs." Chicago: NBC (Television News Report), May 8, 2001.

Bailar, J. "The powerful placebo and the Wizard of Oz." *N Engl J Med* 344, no. 21 (2001): 1630–2.

Bland, J. S. *May 2001 Functional Medicine Update* 21, no.5, Gig Harbor, WA.

Brown, W. A. "The Placebo Effect." *Scientific American*, January, 1998, 90-95.

"Diet and Exercise Sharply Reduce Risk of Adult-Onset Diabetes." *Reuters Medical News*, August 8, 2001.

Graham, N., Burrell, C., Douglas, R., Debelle, P., and Davies, L. "Adverse effects of aspirin, acetaminophen, and ibuprofen on immune function, viral shedding, and clinical status in rhinovirus-infected volunteers." *J Infect Dis* 162, no. 6 (1990): 1277–82.

Hrobjartsson, A., and Gotzsche, P. "Is the placebo powerless? An analysis of clinical trials comparing placebo with no treatment." *N Engl J Med* 344, no. 21 (2001): 1594–602.

Kaushal, R., Bates, D., Landrigan, C., McKenna, K., Clapp, M., Federico, F., and Goldmann, D. "Medication errors and adverse drug events in pediatric inpatients." *JAMA* 285, no. 16 (2001): 2114–20.

Kernan, W., Viscoli, C., Brass, L., Broderick, J., Brott, T., Feldmann, E., Morgenstern, L., Wilterdink, J., and Horwitz, R. "Phenylpropanolamine and the risk of hemorrhagic stroke." *N Engl J Med* 343, no. 25 (2000): 1826–32.

Lazarou, J., Pomeranz, B., and Corey, P. "Incidence of adverse drug reactions in hospitalized patients: a meta-analysis of prospective studies." *JAMA* 279, no. 15 (1998): 1200–5.

Materson, B., Reda, D., Cushman, W., Massie, B., Freis, E., Kochar, M., Hamburger, R., Fye, C., Lakshman, R., Gottdiener, J. , et al. "Single-drug therapy for hypertension in men. A comparison of six antihypertensive agents with placebo. The Department of Veterans Affairs Cooperative Study Group on Antihypertensive Agents." *N Engl J Med* 328, no. 13 (1993): 914–21.

Medical News titled "Walking, Diet Can Cut Diabetes." *Associated Press*, August 8, 2001.

NIH Report titled "Prescription Drug Expenditures in 2000. National Institute for Health Care Management Research and Educational Foundation, Washington, D. C., May, 2001, 1–24.

Report number 0003-9926. Advocates for Highway and Auto Safety, 2001, 0003–9926.

Ricks, D. "Medication Mistakes More Likely in Kids." *Newsday*, April 25, 2001.

Shivkumar, K., Schultz, L., Goldstein, S., and Gheorghiade, M. "Effects of Propanolol in patients entered in the Beta-Blocker Heart Attack Trial with their first myocardial infarction and persistent electro-cardiographic ST-segment depression." *Am Heart J* 135, no. 2 Pt 1 (1998): 261–7.

Shute, N. "Prescribed Killers." *US News and World Report*, April 27, 1998, 71.

Smith, M. "Medicating Kids." *Frontline*, ed. M. Gaviria. Boston: WGBH Boston, 2001.

Thomas, R. "Better drugs, but bigger bills." *The Seattle Times*, March 18, 2001, A1, A25.

Chapter 4

Aldoori, W. "Obesity in developing nations and US weight guidelines [letter; comment]." *JAMA* 274, no. 7 (1995): 537.

Ames, B. "Ames agrees with mom's advice: eat your fruits and vegetables [interview]." *JAMA* 273, no. 14 (1995): 1077–8.

Ames, B. "DNA damage from micronutrient deficiencies is likely to be a major cause of cancer." *Mutation Research* 475, no. 1–2 (2001): 7–20.

Ames, B., Shigenaga, M., and Hagen, T. "Oxidants, antioxidants, and the degenerative diseases of aging." *Proc Natl Acad Sci U S A* 90, no. 17 (1993): 7915–22.

Begley, S. "Stop Blaming Your Genes." *Newsweek*, July 2, 2000, 53.

Block, G., Patterson, B., and Subar, A. "Fruit, vegetables, and cancer prevention: a review of the epidemiological evidence." *Nutr Cancer* 18, no. 1 (1992): 1–29.

Carper, J. "Modern Stone Age Food." *USA WEEKEND*, May 1–3, 1998, 24.

Eaton, S. "Paleolithic vs. modern diets—selected pathophysiological implications." *Eur J Nutr* 39, no. 2 (2000): 67–70.

Fabsitz, R., Carmelli, D., and Hewitt, J. "Evidence for independent genetic influences on obesity in middle age." *Int J Obes Relat Metab Disord* 16, no. 9 (1992): 657–66.

Gibbs, W. W. "Gaining on Fat." *Scientific American*, August, 1996.

Lichtenstein, P., Holm, N., Verkasalo, P., Iliadou, A., Kaprio, J., Koskenvuo, M., Pukkala, E., Skytthe, A., and Hemminki, K. "Environmental and heritable factors in the causation of cancer—analyses of cohorts of twins from Sweden, Denmark, and Finland." *N Engl J Med* 343, no. 2 (2000): 78–85.

Malins, D., Polissar, N., Schaefer, S., Su, Y., and Vinson, M. "A unified theory of carcinogenesis based on order-disorder transitions in DNA structure as studied in the human ovary and breast." *Proc Natl Acad Sci U S A* 95, no. 13 (1998): 7637–42.

Markesbery, W. "The role of oxidative stress in Alzheimer disease." *Arch Neurol* 56, no. 12 (1999): 1449–52.

Marwick, C. "Promising vaccine treatment for alzheimer disease found [news]." *JAMA* 284, no. 12 (2000): 1503–5.

Miranda, S., Opazo, C., Larrondo, L., Munoz, F., Ruiz, F., Leighton, F., and Inestrosa, N. "The role of oxidative stress in the toxicity induced by amyloid beta-peptide in Alzheimer's disease." *Prog Neurobiol* 62, no. 6 (2000): 633–48.

Morgan, D., Diamond, D., Gottschall, P., Ugen, K., Dickey, C., Hardy, J., Duff, K., Jantzen, P., Di, C. G., Wilcock, D. , et al. "A beta peptide vaccination prevents memory loss in an animal model of Alzheimer's disease." *Nature* 408, no. 6815 (2000): 982–5.

Paulson, T. "Seattle biochemist challenging cancer theories." *Seattle Post-Intelligencer*, November 26, 1996, A6.

Ravussin, E. "Effects of a traditional lifestyle on obesity in Pima Indians." *Diabetes Care* 17, no. 9 (1994): 1067–1074.

Varadarajan, S., Yatin, S., Aksenova, M., and Butterfield, D. "Review: Alzheimer's amyloid beta-peptide-associated free radical oxidative stress and neurotoxicity." *J Struct Biol* 130, no. 2–3 (2000): 184–208.

Witte, K., Clark, A., and Cleland, J. "Chronic heart failure and micronutrients." *Journal of the American College of Cardiology* 37, no. 7 (2001): 1765–1774.

Chapter 5

3R's in the Home. The Recycling Council of Ontario, January 10, 2001. Accessed 2001. Internet. Available from: http://www.rco.on.ca/factsheet/3RHome.html

Benzene. Agency for Toxic Substances and Disease Registry Public Health Statement, 1989.

Chloroform. Agency for Toxic Substances and Disease Registry Public Health Statement, 1989.

Cook, D., Shaper, A., Pocock, S., and Kussick, S. "Giving up smoking and the risk of heart attacks. A report from The British Regional Heart Study." *Lancet* 2, no. 8520 (1986): 1376–80.

Doyle, P., Roman, E., Beral, V., and Brookes, M. "Spontaneous abortion in dry cleaning workers potentially exposed to perchloroethylene." *Occup Environ Med* 54, no. 12 (1997): 848–53.

Ott, W. R., and Roberts, J. W. "Everyday Exposure to Toxic Pollutants." *Scientific American*, February, 1998, 86–91.

Wallace, L. A. "Human Exposure to Environmental Pollutants: A Decade of Experience." *Clinical and Experimental Allergy* 25 (1995.): 4–9.

Whitmore, R., Immerman, F., Camann, D., Bond, A., and Lewis, R. "Non-occupational exposure to pesticides for residents of two U.S. cities." *Archives of Environmental Contamination and Toxicology* 26, no. 1 (1994): 47–59.

Zinkernagel, R. M. "Maternal Antibodies, Childhood Infections, and Autoimmune Diseases." *N Engl J Med* 345, no. 18 (2001): 1331–1335.

Chapter 6

Aluminum. Agency for Toxic Substances and Disease Registry, 1995.

Bishop, N., Morley, R., Day, J., and Lucas, A. "Aluminum neurotoxicity in preterm infants receiving intravenous-feeding solutions." *N Engl J Med* 336, no. 22 (1997): 1557–61.

Blaylock, R. "Phytonutrients and metabolic stimulants as protection against neurodegeneration and excitotoxicity." *Journal of the American Nutraceutical Association* 2, no. 3 (2000): 30–39.

Brown-Beasley, M. "After fen-phen/Redux: cardiac and pulmonary sequelae implications for patient assessment." *J Emerg Nurs* 24, no. 1 (1998): 62–5.

Colon, I., Caro, D., Bourdony, C., and Rosario, O. "Identification of phthalate esters in the serum of young Puerto Rican girls with premature breast development." *Environ Health Perspect* 108, no. 9 (2000): 895–900.

Fremerman, S. "Driven to Devour." *Natural Health*, March, 2000, 77–79.

Worldwatch News Release titled "Chronic Hunger and Obesity Epidemic Eroding Global Progress." March 04, 2000. Accessed 2000. Available from: http://www.worldwatch.org/alerts/000304.html

Lemonick, M. D. "Teens Before Their Time." *Time*, October 30, 2000, 66–74.

Page, B., and Lacroix, G. "The occurrence of phthalate ester and di-2-ethylhexyl adipate plasticizers in Canadian packaging and food sampled in 1985–1989: a survey." *Food Addit Contam* 12, no. 1 (1995): 129–51.

Petit, F., Mitz, V., and Chevallier, J. "Morbid obesity: laparoscopic gastroplasty prior to plastic surgery." *Ann Chir* 125, no. 3 (2000): 263–8.

Pottenger Jr., F. M. *Pottenger's Cats*, ed. E. Pottenger and R. T. Pottenger Jr., San Diego: Price-Pottenger Nutrition Foundation, Inc., 1995.

Zinkernagel, R. M. "Maternal Antibodies, Childhood Infections, and Autoimmune Diseases." *N Engl J Med* 345, no. 18 (2001): 1331–1335.

Chapter 7

Ames, B., Shigenaga, M., and Hagen, T. "Oxidants, antioxidants, and the degenerative diseases of aging." *Proc Natl Acad Sci U S A* 90, no. 17 (1993): 7915–22.

Bailar, J. R., and Gornik, H. "Cancer undefeated." *N Engl J Med* 336, no. 22 (1997): 1569–74.

Barker, D. "The fetal origins of coronary heart disease." *Acta Paediatr Suppl* 422 (1997): 78–82.

Begley, S. "Shaped by life in the womb." *Newsweek*, September 27, 1999, 50–57.

Cameron, J., Rosenthal, A., and Olson, A. "Malnutrition in hospitalized children with congenital heart disease." *Arch Pediatr Adolesc Med* 149, no. 10 (1995): 1098–102.

Chen, G., Chung, J., Hsieh, C., and Lin, J. "Effects of the garlic components diallyl sulfide and diallyl disulfide on arylamine N-acetyltransferase activity in human colon tumour cells." *Food Chem Toxicol* 36, no. 9–10 (1998): 761–70.

Chung, J. "Effects of garlic components diallyl sulfide and diallyl disulfide on arylamine N-acetyltransferase activity in human bladder tumor cells." *Drug Chem Toxicol* 22, no. 2 (1999): 343–58.

Furlow, F., Armijo-Prewitt, T., Gangestad, S., and Thornhill, R. "Fluctuating asymmetry and psychometric intelligence." *Proc R Soc Lond B Biol Sci* 264, no. 1383 (1997): 823–9.

Haenlein, G. F., and Ace, D. L. *Extension Goat Handbook.* Washington, D.C.: United States Department of Agriculture Extension Service, 1984, E-1.

Han, S., Chung, S., Robertson, D., Ranjan, D., and Bondada, S. "Curcumin causes the growth arrest and apoptosis of B cell lymphoma by downregulation of egr-1, c-myc, bcl-XL, NF-kappa B, and p53." *Clin Immunol* 93, no. 2 (1999): 152–61.

Huang, C., Ma, W., Goranson, A., and Dong, Z. "Resveratrol suppresses cell transformation and induces apoptosis through a p53-dependent pathway." *Carcinogenesis* 20, no. 2 (1999): 237–42.

Jiang, M., Yang-Yen, H., Yen, J., and Lin, J. "Curcumin induces apoptosis in immortalized NIH 3T3 and malignant cancer cell lines." *Nutr Cancer* 26, no. 1 (1996): 111–20.

Koletzko, B., and Rodriguez-Palmero, M. "Polyunsaturated fatty acids in human milk and their role in early infant development." *J Mammary Gland Biol Neoplasia* 4, no. 3 (1999): 269–84.

Kuo, M., Huang, T., and Lin, J. "Curcumin, an antioxidant and antitumor promoter, induces apoptosis in human leukemia cells." *Biochim Biophys Acta* 1317, no. 2 (1996): 95–100.

Langley-Evans, S., Phillips, G., Benediktsson, R., Gardner, D., Edwards, C., Jackson, A., and Seckl, J. "Protein intake in pregnancy, placental glucocorticoid metabolism and the programming of hypertension in the rat." *Placenta* 17, no. 2–3 (1996): 169–72.

Leeds, A. R., Ferris, E. A. E., Staley, J., Ayesh, R., and Ross, F. "Availability of micronutrients from dried, encapsulated fruit and vegetable preparations: a study in healthy volunteers." *J Hum Nutr Dietet* 13 (2000): 21–27.

Leon, D., Koupilova, I., Lithell, H., Berglund, L., Mohsen, R., Vagero, D., Lithell, U., and McKeigue, P. "Failure to realize growth potential in utero and adult obesity in relation to blood pressure in 50 year old Swedish men." *BMJ* 312, no. 7028 (1996): 401–6.

Lichtenstein, P., Holm, N., Verkasalo, P., Iliadou, A., Kaprio, J., Koskenvuo, M., Pukkala, E., Skytthe, A., and Hemminki, K. "Environmental and heritable factors in the causation of cancer—analyses of cohorts of twins from Sweden, Denmark, and Finland." *N Engl J Med* 343, no. 2 (2000): 78–85.

Lin, J., Chen, Y., Huang, Y., and Lin-Shiau, S. "Suppression of protein kinase C and nuclear oncogene expression as possible molecular mechanisms of cancer chemoprevention by apigenin and curcumin." *J Cell Biochem Suppl* 28–29 (1997): 39–48.

Lingas, R., Dean, F., and Matthews, S. "Maternal nutrient restriction (48 h) modifies brain corticosteroid receptor expression and endocrine function in the fetal guinea pig." *Brain Res* 846, no. 2 (1999): 236–42.

Lithell, H., McKeigue, P., Berglund, L., Mohsen, R., Lithell, U., and Leon, D. "Relation of size at birth to non-insulin dependent diabetes and insulin concentrations in men aged 50–60 years." *BMJ* 312, no. 7028 (1996): 406–10.

Man, W., Weber, M., Palmer, A., Schneider, G., Wadda, R., Jaffar, S., Mulholland, E., and Greenwood, B. "Nutritional status of children admitted to hospital with different diseases and its relationship to outcome in The Gambia, West Africa." *Trop Med Int Health* 3, no. 8 (1998): 678–86.

Michels, K., Trichopoulos, D., Robins, J., Rosner, B., Manson, J., Hunter, D., Colditz, G., Hankinson, S., Speizer, F., and Willett, W. "Birthweight as a risk factor for breast cancer." *Lancet* 348, no. 9041 (1996): 1542–6.

Neugebauer, R., Hoek, H., and Susser, E. "Prenatal exposure to wartime famine and development of antisocial personality disorder in early adulthood." *JAMA* 282, no. 5 (1999): 455–62.

Novak, V. "New Ritalin Ad Blitz Makes Parents Jumpy." *Time* 158, no.10 September 10, 2001.

Potter, J., Klipstein, K., Reilly, J., and Roberts, M. "The nutritional status and clinical course of acute admissions to a geriatric unit." *Age Ageing* 24, no. 2 (1995): 131–6.

Sakamoto, K., Lawson, L., and Milner, J. "Allyl sulfides from garlic suppress the in vitro proliferation of human A549 lung tumor cells." *Nutr Cancer* 29, no. 2 (1997): 152–6.

Seckl, J. "Physiologic programming of the fetus." *Clin Perinatol* 25, no. 4 (1998): 939–62, vii.

Smith, M. J., Inserra, P. F., Watson, R. R., Wise, J. A., and O'Neill, K. L. "Supplementation with fruit and vegetable extracts may decrease DNA damage in the peripheral lymphocytes of an elderly population." *Nutrition Research* 19 (1999): 1507–1518.

Surh, Y., Lee, R., Park, K., Mayne, S., Liem, A., and Miller, J. "Chemoprotective effects of capsaicin and diallyl sulfide against mutagenesis or tumorigenesis by vinyl carbamate and N-nitrosodimethylamine." *Carcinogenesis* 16, no. 10 (1995): 2467–71.

Susser, E., and Lin, S. "Schizophrenia after prenatal exposure to the Dutch Hunger Winter of 1944–1945." *Arch Gen Psychiatry* 49, no. 12 (1992): 983–8.

Weinberg, R. A. "How Cancer Arises." *Scientific American*, September, 1996.

Wise, J. A., Morin, R. J., Sanderson, R., and Blum, K. "Changes in plasma carotenoid, alpha-tocopherol, and lipid peroxide levels in response to supplementation with concentrated fruit and vegetable extracts: a pilot study." *Current Therapeutic Research* 57 (1996): 445–461.

Yuan, F., Chen, D., Liu, K., Sepkovic, D., Bradlow, H., and Auborn, K. "Anti-estrogenic activities of indole-3-carbinol in cervical cells: implication for prevention of cervical cancer." *Anticancer Res* 19, no. 3A (1999): 1673–80.

Chapter 8

Ames, B., Shigenaga, M., and Hagen, T. "Oxidants, antioxidants, and the degenerative diseases of aging." *Proc Natl Acad Sci U S A* 90, no. 17 (1993): 7915–22.

Appel, L., Moore, T., Obarzanek, E., Vollmer, W., Svetkey, L., Sacks, F., Bray, G., Vogt, T., Cutler, J., Windhauser, M. , et al. "A clinical trial of the effects of dietary patterns on blood pressure. DASH Collaborative Research Group." *N Engl J Med* 336, no. 16 (1997): 1117–24.

Coquette, A., Vray, B., and Vanderpas, J. "Role of vitamin E in the protection of the resident macrophage membrane against oxidative damage." *Arch Int Physiol Biochim* 94, no. 5 (1986): S29–34.

Di, C. M. M., de, B. V., Vale, M., and Viana, G. "Lipid peroxidation and nitrite plus nitrate levels in brain tissue from patients with Alzheimer's disease." *Gerontology* 46, no. 4 (2000): 179–84.

Inserra, P. F., Jiang, S., Solkoff, D., Lee, J., Zhang, Z., Xu, M., Hesslink, R., Wise, J. A., and Watson, R. R. "Immune function in elderly smokers and nonsmokers improves during supplementation with fruit and vegetable extracts." *Integrative Medicine* 2, no. 1 (1999): 3–10.

Lisitsyna, T., Ivanova, M., and Durnev, A. "Active forms of oxygen and pathogenesis of rheumatoid arthritis and systemic lupus erythematosus." *Vestn Ross Akad Med Nauk*, no. 12 (1996): 15–20.

Mortensen, E., Jensen, H., Sanders, S., and Reinisch, J. "Better psychological functioning and higher social status may largely explain the apparent health benefits of wine: a study of wine and beer drinking in young Danish adults." *Arch Intern Med* 161, no. 15 (2001): 1844–8.

Papas, A. M. "Antioxidant status, diet, nutrition and health." In *CRC Series in Contemporary Food Science*, 650. Boca Raton: CRC Press, 1999.

Rahman, I., Morrison, D., Donaldson, K., and MacNee, W. "Systemic oxidative stress in asthma, COPD, and smokers." *Am J Respir Crit Care Med* 154, no. 4 Pt 1 (1996): 1055–60.

Sayre, L., Zelasko, D., Harris, P., Perry, G., Salomon, R., and Smith, M. "4-Hydroxynonenal-derived advanced lipid peroxidation end products are increased in Alzheimer's disease." *J Neurochem* 68, no. 5 (1997): 2092–7.

Singh, R., Niaz, M., Agarwal, P., Begom, R., and Rastogi, S. "Effect of antioxidant-rich foods on plasma ascorbic acid, cardiac enzyme, and lipid peroxide levels in patients hospitalized with acute myocardial infarction." *J Am Diet Assoc* 95, no. 7 (1995): 775–80.

Steinberg, D., Parthasarathy, S., Carew, T., Khoo, J., and Witztum, J. "Beyond cholesterol. Modifications of low-density lipoprotein that increase its atherogenicity." *N Engl J Med* 320, no. 14 (1989): 915–24.

Thompson, H., Heimendinger, J., Haegele, A., Sedlacek, S., Gillette, C., O'Neill, C., Wolfe, P., and Conry, C. "Effect of increased vegetable and fruit consumption on markers of oxidative cellular damage." *Carcinogenesis* 20, no. 12 (1999): 2261–6.

Weindruch, R., and Sohal, R. "Seminars in medicine of the Beth Israel Deaconess Medical Center. Caloric intake and aging." *N Engl J Med* 337, no. 14 (1997): 986–94.

Willett, W. *Eat, Drink and Be Healthy.* New York: Simon & Schuster Source, 2001, 134–5.

Wise, J. A., Morin, R. J., Sanderson, R., and Blum, K. "Changes in plasma carotenoid, alpha-tocopherol, and lipid peroxide levels in response to supplementation with concentrated fruit and vegetable extracts: a pilot study." *Current Therapeutic Research* 57 (1996): 445–461.

Chapter 9

Ames, M. "Nourishing Mother and Fetus." *International Journal of Integrative Medicine* Vol. 1, no. No. 6 (1999).

Babbs, C., and Steiner, M. "Simulation of free radical reactions in biology and medicine: a new two-compartment kinetic model of intracellular lipid peroxidation." *Free Radic Biol Med* 8, no. 5 (1990): 471–85.

Balch, J. F., and Balch, P. A. *Prescription for nutritional healing: a practical A to Z reference to drug-free remedies using vitamins, minerals, herbs and food supplements.* 2nd ed. Garden City, New York: Avery Publishing Group, 1997, 7–8.

Cancer study titled "The effect of vitamin E and beta carotene on the incidence of lung cancer and other cancers in male smokers. The Alpha-Tocopherol, Beta Carotene Cancer Prevention Study Group." *N Engl J Med* 330, no. 15 (1994): 1029–35.

Chart titled "Top U.S. Vitamin Manufacturing & Marketing Companies." In *Nutrition Business Journal*, San Diego, 1998.

Hoag, S., Ramachandruni, H., and Shangraw, R. "Failure of prescription prenatal vitamin products to meet USP standards for folic acid dissolution." *J Am Pharm Assoc (Wash)* NS37, no. 4 (1997): 397–400.

Johnson, M., Smith, M., and Edmonds, J. "Copper, iron, zinc, and manganese in dietary supplements, infant formulas, and ready-to-eat breakfast cereals." *Am J Clin Nutr* 67, no. 5 Suppl (1998): 1035S–1040S.

Micozzi, M., Brown, E., Edwards, B., Bieri, J., Taylor, P., Khachik, F., Beecher, G., and Smith, J. J. "Plasma carotenoid response to chronic intake of selected foods and beta-carotene supplements in men." *Am J Clin Nutr* 55, no. 6 (1992): 1120–5.

Newman, V., Lyon, R., and Anderson, P. "Evaluation of prenatal vitamin-mineral supplements." *Clin Pharm* 6, no. 10 (1987): 770–7.

NIH consensus statement titled "Optimal Calcium Intake" June 6–8 1994, 12(4): 1–31 Accessed 2000. Available from: http://text.nlm.nih.gov/nih/cdc/www/97txt.html#Head11

Niki, E., Noguchi, N., Tsuchihashi, H., and Gotoh, N. "Interaction among vitamin C, vitamin E, and beta-carotene." *Am J Clin Nutr* 62, no. 6 Suppl (1995): 1322S–1326S.

O'Brien, K., Zavaleta, N., Caulfield, L., Wen, J., and Abrams, S. "Prenatal iron supplements impair zinc absorption in pregnant Peruvian women." *J Nutr* 130, no. 9 (2000): 2251–5.

Papas, A. M. "Antioxidant status, diet, nutrition and health." In *CRC Series in Contemporary Food Science*, 650. Boca Raton: CRC Press, 1999, 93 & 18.

Stamatakis, M., and Meyer-Stout, P. "Disintegration performance of renal multivitamin supplements." *J Ren Nutr* 9, no. 2 (1999): 78–83.

Stone, W., and Papas, A. "Tocopherols and the etiology of colon cancer." *J Natl Cancer Inst* 89, no. 14 (1997): 1006–14.

Wise, J. A., Morin, R. J., Sanderson, R., and Blum, K. "Changes in plasma carotenoid, alpha-tocopherol, and lipid peroxide levels in response to supplementation with concentrated fruit and vegetable extracts: a pilot study." *Current Therapeutic Research* 57 (1996): 445–461.

Chapter 10

McCullough, M., Feskanich, D., Rimm, E., Giovannucci, E., Ascherio, A., Variyam, J., Spiegelman, D., Stampfer, M., and Willett, W. "Adherence to the Dietary Guidelines for Americans and risk of major chronic disease in men." *Am J Clin Nutr* 72, no. 5 (2000): 1223–31

Schwarzbein, D., and Deville, N. *The Schwarzbein Principle: The Truth About Losing Weight, Being Healthy and Feeling Younger.* Deerfield Beach, FL: Health Communications, Inc., 1999, 50–51.

Chapter 11

American Heart Association position: Accessed 2001. Available from: http://www.americanheart.org/Heart_and_Stroke_A_Z_Guide/fish.html

Biagi, P., Bordoni, A., Hrelia, S., Celadon, M., and Horrobin, D. "Gamma-linolenic acid dietary supplementation can reverse the aging influence on rat liver microsome delta 6-desaturase activity." *Biochim Biophys Acta* 1083, no. 2 (1991): 187–92.

Blonk, M., Bilo, H., Nauta, J., Popp-Snijders, C., Mulder, C., and Donker, A. "Dose-response effects of fish-oil supplementation in healthy volunteers." *Am J Clin Nutr* 52, no. 1 (1990): 120–7.

Bolton-Smith, C., Woodward, M., and Tavendale, R. "Evidence for age-related differences in the fatty acid composition of human adipose tissue, independent of diet." *Eur J Clin Nutr* 51, no. 9 (1997): 619–24.

Byrnes, S. *The Myths of Vegetarianism.* Townsend Letter for Doctors and Patients, Accessed 2001. Available from: http://tldp.com/issue/11_00/veretarianism.html

Carper, J. "Eat Smart: From the fat front." *USA Weekend*, March 3, 2001.

Cook, D., Shaper, A., Pocock, S., and Kussick, S. "Giving up smoking and the risk of heart attacks. A report from The British Regional Heart Study." *Lancet* 2, no. 8520 (1986): 1376–80.

Crawford, M., Gale, M., and Woodford, M. "Linoleic acid and linolenic acid elongation products in muscle tissue of Sncerus caffer and other ruminant species." *Biochem J* 115, no. 1 (1969): 25–7.

Das, U. "Beneficial effect(s) of n-3 fatty acids in cardiovascular diseases: but, why and how?" *Prostaglandins Leukot Essent Fatty Acids* 63, no. 6 (2000): 351–62.

Fallon, S., and Enig, M. G. "Tragedy and Hope: The Third International Soy Symposium—Part I." *Townsend Letter*, July, 2000, 65–71.

Fish oil study titled "Dietary supplementation with n-3 polyunsaturated fatty acids and vitamin E after myocardial infarction: results of the GISSI-Prevenzione trial. Gruppo Italiano per lo Studio della Sopravvivenza nell'Infarto miocardico." *Lancet* 354, no. 9177 (1999): 447–55.

Fremont, L., Belguendouz, L., and Delpal, S. "Antioxidant activity of resveratrol and alcohol-free wine polyphenols related to LDL oxidation and polyunsaturated fatty acids." *Life Sci* 64, no. 26 (1999): 2511–21.

Gillman, M., Cupples, L., Gagnon, D., Millen, B., Ellison, R., and Castelli, W. "Margarine intake and subsequent coronary heart disease in men." *Epidemiology* 8, no. 2 (1997): 144–9.

Haenlein, G. F., and Ace, D. L. *Extension Goat Handbook.* Washington, D.C.: United States Department of Agriculture Extension Service, 1984, E-1.

Haney, D. "Study: Cholesterol-lowering drug may dull your edge." *Associated Press*, November 10, 1997.

Hayashi, Y., and Nakamura, H. "The optimum serum cholesterol level. Preface." *Rinsho Byori* 39, no. 5 (1991): 481–2.

Hjermann, I., Velve, B. K., Holme, I., and Leren, P. "Effect of diet and smoking intervention on the incidence of coronary heart disease. Report from the Oslo Study Group of a randomised trial in healthy men." *Lancet* 2, no. 8259 (1981): 1303–10.

Hornstra, G. "Essential fatty acids in mothers and their neonates." *Am J Clin Nutr* 71, no. 5 Suppl (2000): 1262S–9S.

Horrobin, D. F. "Fatty acid metabolism in health and disease: the role of delta-6-desaturase." *Am J Clin Nutr* 57, no. 5 Suppl (1993): 732S–736S.

Jordan, K. G. "Fats for Life." *Life Extension* (2001): 20–32.

Kannel, W., and Gordon, T. "The search for an optimum serum cholesterol." *Lancet* 2, no. 8294 (1982): 374–5.

Kirschenbauer, H. G. *Fats and oils: an outline of their chemistry and technology.* 2d ed. New York,: Reinhold Pub. Corp., 1960.

Kochetova, M., Eremina, I., Kliuchnikova, Z., Solov'eva, E., Butusova, N., Torkhovskaia, T., and Khalilov, E. "[The antiatherogenic action of plant oils with added omega-3 polyunsaturated fatty acids]." *Biull Eksp Biol Med* 116, no. 10 (1993): 407–9.

Kushi, L., Folsom, A., Prineas, R., Mink, P., Wu, Y., and Bostick, R. "Dietary antioxidant vitamins and death from coronary heart disease in postmenopausal women." *N Engl J Med* 334, no. 18 (1996): 1156–62.

Kwak, B., Mulhaupt, F., Myit, S., and Mach, F. "Statins as a newly recognized type of immunomodulator." *Nat Med* 6, no. 12 (2000): 1399–402.

Liu, S., Willett, W., Stampfer, M., Hu, F., Franz, M., Sampson, L., Hennekens, C., and Manson, J. "A prospective study of dietary glycemic load, carbohydrate intake, and risk of coronary heart disease in US women." *Am J Clin Nutr* 71, no. 6 (2000): 1455–61.

Papas, A. M. "Antioxidant status, diet, nutrition and health." In *CRC Series in Contemporary Food Science*, 650. Boca Raton: CRC Press, 1999, 73–74.

Plotnick, G., Corretti, M., and Vogel, R. "Effect of antioxidant vitamins on the transient impairment of endothelium-dependent brachial artery vasoactivity following a single high-fat meal." *JAMA* 278, no. 20 (1997): 1682–6.

Plotnick, G., Corretti, M., Vogel, R., Hesslink, R., Balon, T., and Wise, J. A. "The effects of supplemental phytonutrients on endothelial function." In *2nd Annual International Congress of Heart Disease — New Trends in Research, Diagnosis and Treatment*, 2. Washington, DC: International Academic Communications, 2001.

Rinzler, C. A. *Nutrition for Dummies.* San Francisco, CA: Hungry Minds, 1999, 28 & 100.

Roberts, S. "High-glycemic index foods, hunger, and obesity: is there a connection?" *Nutr Rev* 58, no. 6 (2000): 163–9.

Schwarzbein, D., and Deville, N. *The Schwarzbein Principle: The Truth About Losing Weight, Being Healthy and Feeling Younger.* Deerfield Beach, FL: Health Communications, Inc., 1999, 80.

Simopoulos, A., and Salem, N. J. "Egg yolk as a source of long-chain polyunsaturated fatty acids in infant feeding." *Am J Clin Nutr* 55, no. 2 (1992): 411–4.

Sternberg, S. "Warning labels urged for cholesterol drugs." *USA TODAY*, 8/20/2001, 2001.

Stryer, L. *Biochemistry.* 3rd ed. New York: W.H. Freeman, 1988, 634.

Suzuki, H., Manabe, S., Wada, O., and Crawford, M. "Rapid incorporation of docosahexaenoic acid from dietary sources into brain microsomal, synaptosomal and mitochondrial membranes in adult mice." *Int J Vitam Nutr Res* 67, no. 4 (1997): 272–8.

Wollschlaeger, B. "Statin Drugs and Coenzyme Q10: A Potential for Drug Nutrient Depletion." *Journal of the American Nutraceutical Association* 4, no. 1 (2001): 7–8.

Youdim, K., Martin, A., and Joseph, J. "Essential fatty acids and the brain: possible health implications." *Int J Dev Neurosci* 18, no. 4–5 (2000): 383–99.

Chapter 12

Atkins, R. C. *Dr. Atkins' New Diet Revolution.* New York: Avon Books, 1999.

Curley, M., and Castillo, L. "Nutrition and shock in pediatric patients." *New Horiz* 6, no. 2 (1998): 212–25.

Evans, W., and Rosenberg, I. H. *Biomarkers—The 10 Keys To Prolonging Vitality.* First ed. New York: Fireside, 1992.

Hellmich, N., "Success of Atkins is in the Calories." USA Today, Oct 29, 2000.

Kaats, G. R., Wise, J. A., Morin, R. J., Pullin, D., Squires, W., and Hesslink, R. "Positive Effects of Nutritional Supplements on Body Composition Biomarkers of Aging During a Weight Loss Program." *Journal of the American Nutraceutical Association* 1, no. 1 (1998): 1–7.

Wise, J. A. "Unpublished 8 week study, 1999." personal communication to M. Ray.

Zinkernagel, R. M. "Maternal Antibodies, Childhood Infections, and Autoimmune Diseases." *N Engl J Med* 345, no. 18 (2001): 1331–1335.

Chapter 13

Cohen, S., Line, S., Manuck, S., Rabin, B., Heise, E., and Kaplan, J. "Chronic social stress, social status, and susceptibility to upper respiratory infections in nonhuman primates." *Psychosom Med* 59, no. 3 (1997): 213–21.

Cohen, S., Tyrrell, D., and Smith, A. "Psychological stress and susceptibility to the common cold." *N Engl J Med* 325, no. 9 (1991): 606–12.

Dallman, M., Akana, S., Strack, A., Hanson, E., and Sebastian, R. "The neural network that regulates energy balance is responsive to glucocorticoids and insulin and also regulates HPA axis responsivity at a site proximal to CRF neurons." *Ann N Y Acad Sci* 771 (1995): 730–42.

Elenkov, I., and Chrousos, G. "Stress, cytokine patterns and susceptibility to disease." *Baillieres Best Pract Res Clin Endocrinol Metab* 13, no. 4 (1999): 583–95.

Liu, D., Diorio, J., Tannenbaum, B., Caldji, C., Francis, D., Freedman, A., Sharma, S., Pearson, D., Plotsky, P., and Meaney, M. "Maternal care, hippocampal glucocorticoid receptors, and hypothalamic-pituitary-adrenal responses to stress." *Science* 277, no. 5332 (1997): 1659–62.

Lundberg, U., and Frankenhaeuser, M. "Stress and workload of men and women in high-ranking positions." *J Occup Health Psychol* 4, no. 2 (1999): 142–51.

McCraty, R., Atkinson, M., Tomasino, D., Goelitz, J., and Mayrovitz, H. "The impact of an emotional self-management skills course on psychosocial functioning and autonomic recovery to stress in middle school children." *Integr Physiol Behav Sci* 34, no. 4 (1999): 246–68.

Sapolsky, R. M. *Why Zebras Don't Get Ulcers.* New York: Freeman, 1999, 264–270.

Chapter 14

Aldoori, W., Giovannucci, E., Rimm, E., Ascherio, A., Stampfer, M., Colditz, G., Wing, A., Trichopoulos, D., and Willett, W. "Prospective study of physical activity and the risk of symptomatic diverticular disease in men." *Gut* 36, no. 2 (1995): 276–82.

Arroll, B., and Beaglehole, R. "Does physical activity lower blood pressure: a critical review of the clinical trials." *J Clin Epidemiol* 45, no. 5 (1992): 439–47.

Ashton, W., Nanchahal, K., and Wood, D. "Leisure-time physical activity and coronary risk factors in women." *J Cardiovasc Risk* 7, no. 4 (2000): 259–66.

Birch, B. B. *Power yoga : the total strength and flexibility workout.* New York: Simon & Schuster, 1995.

Blumenthal, J., Babyak, M., Moore, K., Craighead, W., Herman, S., Khatri, P., Waugh, R., Napolitano, M., Forman, L., Appelbaum, M., et al. "Effects of exercise training on older patients with major depression." *Arch Intern Med* 159, no. 19 (1999): 2349–56.

Campbell, A., Robertson, M., Gardner, M., Norton, R., Tilyard, M., and Buchner, D. "Randomised controlled trial of a general practice programme of home based exercise to prevent falls in elderly women." *BMJ* 315, no. 7115 (1997): 1065–9.

Ettinger, W., Burns, R., Messier, S., Applegate, W., Rejeski, W., Morgan, T., Shumaker, S., Berry, M., O'Toole, M., Monu, J., et al. "A randomized trial comparing aerobic exercise and resistance exercise with a health education program in older adults with knee osteoarthritis. The Fitness Arthritis and Seniors Trial (FAST)." *JAMA* 277, no. 1 (1997): 25–31.

Evans, W., and Rosenberg, I. H. *Biomarkers—The 10 Keys To Prolonging Vitality.* First ed. New York: Fireside, 1992, 14.

Fenton, M., and Feury, M. "Commit 2B Fit." *Walking,* October, 2000, 70–75.

Garfinkel, M., Singhal, A., Katz, W., Allan, D., Reshetar, R., and Schumacher, H. "Yoga-based intervention for carpal tunnel syndrome: a randomized trial." *JAMA* 280, no. 18 (1998): 1601–3.

Giovannucci, E., Ascherio, A., Rimm, E., Colditz, G., Stampfer, M., and Willett, W. "Physical activity, obesity, and risk for colon cancer and adenoma in men." *Ann Intern Med* 122, no. 5 (1995): 327–34.

Hu, F., Sigal, R., Rich-Edwards, J., Colditz, G., Solomon, C., Willett, W., Speizer, F., and Manson, J. "Walking compared with vigorous physical activity and risk of type 2 diabetes in women: a prospective study." *JAMA* 282, no. 15 (1999): 1433–9.

Katzmarzyk, P., Gagnon, J., Leon, A., Skinner, J., Wilmore, J., Rao, D., and Bouchard, C. "Fitness, fatness, and estimated coronary heart disease risk: the HERITAGE Family Study." *Med Sci Sports Exerc* 33, no. 4 (2001): 585–90.

King, A., Oman, R., Brassington, G., Bliwise, D., and Haskell, W. "Moderate-intensity exercise and self-rated quality of sleep in older adults. A randomized controlled trial." *JAMA* 277, no. 1 (1997): 32–7.

Leitzmann, M., Rimm, E., Willett, W., Spiegelman, D., Grodstein, F., Stampfer, M., Colditz, G., and Giovannucci, E. "Recreational physical activity and the risk of cholecystectomy in women." *N Engl J Med* 341, no. 11 (1999): 777–84.

Malathi, A., and Damodaran, A. "Stress due to exams in medical students—role of yoga." *Indian J Physiol Pharmacol* 43, no. 2 (1999): 218–24.

Manchanda, S., Narang, R., Reddy, K., Sachdeva, U., Prabhakaran, D., Dharmanand, S., Rajani, M., and Bijlani, R. "Retardation of coronary atherosclerosis with yoga lifestyle intervention." *J Assoc Physicians India* 48, no. 7 (2000): 687–94.

Manjunath, N., and Telles, S. "Factors influencing changes in tweezer dexterity scores following yoga training." *Indian J Physiol Pharmacol* 43, no. 2 (1999): 225–9.

Manson, J., Hu, F., Rich-Edwards, J., Colditz, G., Stampfer, M., Willett, W., Speizer, F., and Hennekens, C. "A prospective study of walking as compared with vigorous exercise in the prevention of coronary heart disease in women." *N Engl J Med* 341, no. 9 (1999): 650–8.

Martinez, M., Giovannucci, E., Spiegelman, D., Hunter, D., Willett, W., and Colditz, G. "Leisure-time physical activity, body size, and colon cancer in women. Nurses' Health Study Research Group." *J Natl Cancer Inst* 89, no. 13 (1997): 948–55.

Platz, E., Kawachi, I., Rimm, E., Colditz, G., Stampfer, M., Willett, W., and Giovannucci, E. "Physical activity and benign prostatic hyperplasia." *Arch Intern Med* 158, no. 21 (1998): 2349–56.

Report titled "Ten Exercise Myths." *Nutrition Action Healthletter*, January/February, 2000.

Report titled "A Dozen Other Reasons to Exercise." *Nutrion Action Health Letter*, January/February, 2000.

Steptoe, A., Edwards, S., Moses, J., and Mathews, A. "The effects of exercise training on mood and perceived coping ability in anxious adults from the general population." *J Psychosom Res* 33, no. 5 (1989): 537–47.

Wang, J., Lan, C., and Wong, M. "Tai Chi Chuan training to enhance microcirculatory function in healthy elderly men." *Arch Phys Med Rehabil* 82, no. 9 (2001): 1176–80.

Wolff, I., van Croonenborg, C. J., Kemper, H., Kostense, P., and Twisk, J. "The effect of exercise training programs on bone mass: a meta-analysis of published controlled trials in pre- and postmenopausal women." *Osteoporos Int* 9, no. 1 (1999): 1–12.

Conclusion

Ames, B. *Micronutrient Deficiencies in Our Diets: Do They Damage DNA? How Do These Deficiencies Impact the Prevention of Cancer and Other Degenerative Diseases Associated with Aging?* San Diego, CA: The American Nutraceutical Association, 2001.

Choi, S., and Mason, J. "Folate and carcinogenesis: an integrated scheme." *J Nutr* 130, no. 2 (2000): 129–32.

Ellithorpe, R. R. "Whole Food Based Nutritional Supplement Increases Antioxidant Levels in the Blood." *Journal of the American Nutraceutical Association* 4, no. 2 (2001): 44–48.

Gorman, C. "Repairing the Damage." *Time*, February 5, 2001.

Hayflick, L. "The future of ageing." *Nature* 408, no. 6809 (2000): 267–9.

PBS series titled "The Adult Brain" episode 4 of *The Secret Life of the Brain* Accessed February 6, 2002. Available from: http://www.pbs.org/wnet/brain/episode4/index.html

Zinkernagel, R. M. "Maternal Antibodies, Childhood Infections, and Autoimmune Diseases." *N Engl J Med* 345, no. 18 (2001): 1331–1335.

Index

vitamins 155, 158, 164, 165, 166, 170, 175, 186, 197, 234, 249, 274, 336
VLDL 208
VO2 max 312
weight loss 263, 264, 265, 266, 268, 269, 272, 273, 284, 311
whole food 189, 197, 198, 209, 217, 222, 236, 274, 281, 284, 308, 309, 310, 336

yoga 311, 312, 314, 315, 316, 319, 321, 322, 324

zinc 159, 160, 165, 169, 170, 246
Zone 177, 178, 196

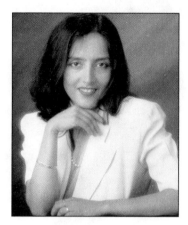

Mitra Ray, Ph.D. is a woman with a mission. She wants each and every one of us to live the longest, healthiest life possible. She believes that in order to do this, we have to be willing to take full responsibility for our health and to begin to apply some fundamental principles of biochemistry and physiology in our daily lives.

As a biochemist with a Ph.D. in cell biology from Stanford University, Dr. Ray has worked in the area of degenerative diseases, such as cancer and Alzheimer's disease—her research funded by the National Institutes of Health, the American Cancer Society and an Alzheimer's Research Grant. But in 1994, Dr. Ray made an important life-altering *personal* discovery that changed her life and her work forever. After trying conventional methods of remedying excruciating back spasms—everything from complete rest to pharmaceutical intervention—Dr. Ray changed her diet, and her back pain subsided. Preventative concepts, such as whole food nutrition, became her new direction in research.

Today Dr. Ray shares what she has learned about prevention with thousands around the world. She has given health seminars to audiences in the United States, Canada and Europe, and has sold over a million copies of her *Fountain of Health* audiotapes.

Dr. Ray and her husband are the proud parents of two lovely, healthy girls.